DECODING THE BRAIN

ISBN 0-9741190-4-0

Biblio Books

Biblio Books Israel, Acco ○ Biblio Books International, Miami
http://www.bibliobooks.com ○email info@bibliobooks.com

I want to thank Dr Billy Reeves, who encouraged me to persist, and Professor Marcela Trevino, who made editing suggestions

Table of Contents

Chapter 1: Introduction

All sensory systems in multicellular animals (metazoans) have non-nerve cells at the body surface (or recessed within that surface) forming discrete "sense organs." Regardless of the form of matter/energy triggering particular "sense organs," the triggered cells transmit bioelectric potentials along peripheral nerves to the spinal cord (or the brain stem in the case of the sensory components of the cranial nerves) to discrete "sensory receptor" regions in the cerebral cortex. In these cortical sensory receptor areas, cerebral neurons (gray brain cells) vary in electrical state when receiving potentials from the periphery. Now, a human red blood cell is, on average, seven microns or seven millionths of a meter in diameter. A meter is 39.37 inches, or slightly longer than a yard. Therefore, roughly 3,629 aligned and contiguous red cells equal one inch. If nerve cells of both peripheral nerves and the brain are of roughly comparable size, then the distance from tactile detectors in the sole of the foot of six foot tall men, to the brain cells triggered in the somesthetic cortex (1.8 meters) contains 257,148 aligned, juxtaposed neurons (in peripheral nerves and spinal cord). Even the distance from humans' retinae, inner ears (cochleae), taste buds or nasal mucosa to their respective cerebral sensory receptor cells contains roughly 43,543 interposed cells, since the pathway length (cranial nerves to brain stem and in some cases upper cervical spinal cord and thence to cerebral sensory receptor neurons) is roughly one foot (1 meter divided by 0.000007 = 142,858 cells/meter, divided by 39.37 inches = 3,629 cells/inch x 12 inches = 43,543 cells/foot). Since cerebral sensory receptor neurons vary in electrical state when stimulated from the periphery regardless of the peripheral sensory detector, then the separation and characterization into distinct sensory modes (tact, olfaction, gustation, sight, hearing, echolocation, remote thermal and remote bioelectric location) must take place in the brain downstream of cerebral sensory receptor neurons varying in response to action potentials from the body surface. Since the only physical resource contained in brains available to measure (compare) variations of electrical state of cerebral neurons is other cerebral neurons, the processes of measurement and analysis must consist of structurally significant and bioelectrically dynamic events involving synaptic links between brain cells (geometrically specific circuits) and the bioelectric peculiarities within and between circuits. Circuit geometry and specific bioelectric events must be symbolically meaningful because the content of consciousness (starting with awareness of the configuration and shape of the body surface, of light, sound and non-body molecules [smell and taste]) does not consist of actual intracerebral anatomic charts, light, sound waves etc. The challenge of understanding (thereby defining) consciousness, how it is elaborated, and in what specific and arbitrary order is the same whether one seeks to explain how we acquire sentience or how the first multicellular animal with a particular sensation (sight, hearing, smell etc) acquired such modality.

Accepting biological evolution by natural selection means acknowledging that life began as single, non-nucleated cells (prokaryotes) some of which evolved to nucleated cells (eukaryotes) some of which evolved into multicellular animals which in turn evolved into invertebrates, vertebrates and the last, into fish, amphibians, reptiles, birds and mammals. Multicellular vertebrates and invertebrates consist of tissues and organs performing specific tasks for the multicellular collective, including detection of body and non-body macroscopic matter/energy. By definition, this collective enterprise is an impossibility for one-celled animals (protozoa). Also by definition, protozoa have no means for "sensing" macroscopic matter and energy. They can neither elaborate nor have awareness of things macroscopic. In metazoans, nervous systems including brains serve to monitor the macroscopic world (which the animal is part of) and maneuver the multicellular being in that world. Every sensory modality (and thus every form of "sensation") emerged for the first time in a first animal equipped to deploy that modality and therefore sensation. This ancestor had no "genetic" knowledge of the phenomenon (light, sound, odors etc). From that point on, DNA assured transmission of the sense organ and its connections to the brain, in the descendants of the sensory Prometheus. DNA cannot, however, transmit the content, or awareness of an aspect of the macro world, which corret and timely functioning of the sensory system and its cerebral analysis make possible. Just as the ancestral first animal with any given sensory system, having no ancestors endowed with that form of sentience, had to elaborate same—, so we, if born with the appropriate organs and with the tracts linking them to our brain, may acquire the "sensation" if the organ is stimulated in early life and the cerebral processing of signals from it is correct. Sensations must form before a deadline age in the young. They do not form after that deadline. Tact, sight, echolocation, remote animal heat location etc. each arose a first time in some vertebrate or invertebrate. The first animal with that "sensation" genetically bequeathed the organ(s), and the tracts linking same with a cerebral "sensory receptor" region, to its descendants. And just as the ancestor first having and deploying the system had no genetic concept of the phenomenon triggering the system, all animals born with it must acquire a symbolic awareness of said phenomenon through correct symbolic, logical and data-averaging cerebral neuronal-circuit operations on signals received from the peripheral detector in early life and this must happen by a deadline age. It is documented that non-correction of defective sensory detectors before a deadline age signifies failure to acquire the "sensation." Thus, cochlear (inner ear) damage-due to infection, for example- is treatable with electronic cochlear implants if performed before the deadline. "Hearing" and the concept of sound can develop. But the identical procedure performed after the deadline leaves sufferers congenitally deaf, with no concept of sound. Similarly, strabismus (cross-eyes) causes non-acquisition of depth perception if untreated. Treated before the deadline age, stereopsis develops. Treated after that age, it does not. Babies with untreated cochlear damage or whose electronic implants were placed too late, never learn spoken language. If the content of awareness were genetically passed on rather than the organs and pathways whose timely triggering and cerebral processing builds consciousness, then we would speak and read our parents' language(s) without schooling, know the science and arts they mastered without schooling etc. And people born with cochlear defects or cross-eyes would require no medical/surgical corrections to know sound and depth perception since their ancestors possessed same. Last, there is documentation that fish and salamanders with sight, which become trapped in lightless caves, give rise after many generations to descendants without eyes. They are blind despite descent from ancestors with sight. The conclusion from all the above is that elaborating consciousness is an active, dynamic and de novo process in each multicellular animal. Since light, non-body pressures, textures and temperature, sound, odors etc are absent in brains, then sensations are symbolic concepts rather than actual lights, sounds and so on. Since the living elements elaborating and forming concepts are cerebral neurons, concepts are symbolic items formed by structural combinations of neurons (circuits) which are symbolic and within and between which, bioelectric events are symbolically meaningful. To recapitulate: Sensory systems composed of multiple, non-neuronal cells organized as detection organs for finite aspects of macroscopic matter/energy located at or within body surfaces and linked by multiple nerve cells to receptor neurons in brains, evolved by natural selection eons after single-celled organisms were the only life forms. Every form of "sensation" found in the contemporary animal kingdom arose in a first animal to possess that sensory system. These first animals had no genetic (inherited) concept of the awareness (i.e. information regarding the macro world) the system can yield. In these animal firsts, the sensation arose through timely triggering of the system, involving a series of symbolic logical and data-averaging operations by and between cerebral neural circuits. Contemporary animals (humans included) do not develop sight, hearing and speech unless their audiovisual systems (at the body surface and in the brain) functioned correctly in infancy. Thus, contemporary fauna must elaborate sensations by a sequence of symbolically logical cerebral neural operations just as did the first animals with a given species' sensory menu. The analytical exercises needed to understand and thus define sensations, perceptions, ideas and Mind are thus identical whether we consider contemporary fauna or ancestral first animals with particular sensations. Invoking genetics to explain the content of awareness rather than the differentiation of cells into peripheral detectors and pathways linking them to the brain, is either a deliberate or unconscious ploy to avoid reasoning out how non-neural detectors of matter/energy, relaying bioelectric potentials to brain cells, culminates in consciousness. Such analysis, or reasoning out, became possible only after nerve cells were identified by silver stains in the 1890s. With this datum, and previously described bioelectricity and cerebral compartmentalization, substituting genetics for analysis of data constitutes intellectual sloth or timidity. An analogous situation obtains in the matter of the origin of life. Here, the challenge is to show how life arose from inert matter and unstructured energy. The "primal soup" hypothesis of Oparin (a mix of amino acids in water presumed to duplicate the early ocean, submitted to electric charges mimicking lightning etc) is an intellectually honest attempt to solve the riddle. Postulating that earthly life arrived on comets or spaceships is avoiding the question of how life arose from non-living matter/energy. It is a non-answer just as genetics explains nothing about the content of consciousness.

Multicellularity: Rationale and Symbolism

Symbols are material constructs agreed by consensus to represent concepts. Flags and anthems stand for nations and sovereignty, skulls and crossed bones for poison and piracy. Non-body phenomena detected by macroscopic "sense organs" are absent in brains. Accordingly, awareness of same is concepts made up of symbolically meaningful structural/dynamic constructs of brain cells and bioelectricity. The symbolism is proper to the brain(s) performing and completing symbolic logical/data-averaging analysis of variations of cerebral "sensory receptor" neurons in response to signals of extra cerebral origin. The symbolism is a necessary result of the evolution of some protozoa into multicellular organisms. What is the rationale for multicellularity?

The cell membrane of protozoans is their principle defense against environmental danger. These dangers, for one-celled microscopic organisms, are themselves of microscopic orders of magnitude: other microorganisms and chemical/energy hazards on a micro scale. The membrane works as a molecular lock and key device, as first understood by professor Paul Ehrlich in the late nineteenth century. Non-cell items of suitable molecular configuration (ideally, food and energy) pass through the membrane while harmful/lethal items are excluded by it. But some harmful/lethal items gain entry by closely resembling the molecular structure of desirable items, like carbon monoxide displacing oxygen in erythrocytes. Yet other phenomena breach or destroy the membrane by brute mechanical force or energy. View these microscopic threats, optimizing survival of one-celled organisms suggests two stratagems. One is rapid unicellular asexual duplication. The odds of meeting, being penetrated and destroyed by germicidal agents is actuarially time-related. Damage/ lethality are, statistically, likely at some minimal time intervals. Survival of protozoan colonies (but not individuals) improves when cells reduplicate at time intervals smaller than the statistically minimal interval likely to result in encountering hazards. This no doubt explains why some protozoa reduplicate every half-hour. The second stratagem is multicellularity. Some cells achieve protection from microscopic hazards through the interposition of multiple other cells constituted into surrounding tissues and organs. Tissues composed of ecto, meso and endoderm evolved to encase and protect selected cells, be they cerebral neurons or sex cells. In the resultant metazoan organism, brains composed of gray (thinking) and white (support and immunologic) cells function to interpret signals about the macroscopic environment received from sense organs, and to command appropriate responses by the multicellular collective. Multicellular animals with brains accordingly have a finite number of sensory systems triggered by finite spectra of non-body macroscopic matter and energy. Mobile metazoans also have a single, peripheral voluntary muscle system enabling displacements in the macro world. Cerebral neurons involved in monitoring that world and maneuvering in it are unaware of things microscopic. The micro world is monitored and responded to by the immune and autonomic nervous systems, and tissues and organs filtering microscopic and molecular items (liver, intestines, lungs). Cortical neurons (archepallium, paleopallium and neopallium or neocortex) produce a functional, logical-symbolic fusion of the finite sensory inputs to, and single muscular output-response of the brain to form a single, coherent whole. This is why we can simultaneously see vehicular traffic and traffic lights, smell automobile exhausts, hear fog horns, taste chewing gum, grasp a briefcase and walk across the street, all seamlessly. It follows that multicellularity requires of the monitoring/response-ordering center of the organism (its brain) certain premises concerning the multicellular body it controls, and the macro world around it. First, is the need to demarcate body from non-body, that is: establishing the boundaries of self. In one-celled animals, that boundary is the cell membrane. But neurons are unaware of themselves, of being cells, and of being situated in brains enclosed in soft tissues (meninges) and bones. They are ignorant of the compartmentalization within brains into regions performing discrete symbolic processing of bioelectricity (which they are ignorant of) or the existence of tracts from peripheral sensors to brains, and from brains to muscles (which they know nothing of). Neurons don't know the gross anatomy nor histology of the tissues and organs constituting the multicellular being they manipulate, nor its internal milieu (viscera, cardiovascular and lymphatic systems) which are regulated by the autonomic nervous system. Fusing macroscopic sensory inputs with muscular output into one coherent whole creates a symbolic neural concept of self. This integration is a must for cerebral neural logical/symbolic processing of intracerebral bioelectric variations. This self or "I" is not that of psychiatry (ego) which is awareness of individuality relative to others of the species. "I" is a logical/mathematical constant needed so that neural circuits may undertake symbolic analysis of intracerebral bioelectrical variations. Brains must have fused Is equal in number to the sensory modalities of the species plus the cerebrally ordered muscle response (active or passive) to the combined sensory inputs. There are two reasons why Is must be fused or integrated. First, to enable the biologic computer (for that is what nervous systems are) to synaptically establish its "I," and second, to avoid autism and schizophrenia (which have got to be a non-fusion of two or more Is). Some might argue that multiple Is necessarily produces schizophrenia. This is belied by contemplation of the forms taken by multicellularity. Even microscopically, there is a model of fusion according to a hypothesis whose chief proponent in

s, there must be an integrative fault where
l analysis and critique is unable to data aver-
nadequate at it. Hallucinations are accepted
value despite other indications that the room
y (hence no voices, monsters, creepy-crawlies,
r tastes).

thus a fusion of sensory inputs and the soli-
tor output of brains, so that all macroscopic
nces are rendered a seamless whole. For this
rialize, "I" must consider a part of the multi-
collective to be the "I"—"non-"I" boundary
oundary, enclosing the totality of "I," is the
kin becomes, accordingly, the fused cerebral
circuits' metaphor for the cell membrane of
ed biota. It is not, actually, the boundary
cerebral neurons and the environment of
ulticellular being, but they are obliged to con-
so , thereby rendering it a logical constant of
bolic monitoring of and maneuvering in the
world. Skin is metazoans' neural metaphor
protozoan cell membrane.

ie protozoa have phototropism, that is their
ng-distance sensory detection modality. All
nicellular "sensations" analogous to meta-
involve direct contact with the cell mem-
Apposition of matter to the membrane equals
n "tactile" sensation and sound detection
causes vibratory waves in water or air, and
pact the membrane whereas it is cochlear
r cells that detect sound in metazoans). Mol-
detected by metazoan nasal and lingual cells
inate in "smell" and "taste") also directly
protozoan cell membranes. Brains, on the

this generation is professor Lynn Margulis. Said hypothesis affirms that some intracellular inclusions in eukaryotes were originally independent microorganisms (ribosomes, mitochondria, endoplasmic reticulum). There was presumably a first stage of symbiosis, and over geologic time spans symbiosis led to fusion, resulting in single-celled biota of some internal complexity. At the multicellular scale, there are clearly cases of symbiosis (e.g. fish living between the tentacles of sea anemones, luring others to the tentacles and feeding on scraps). There is a mutually beneficial relationship with retention of individuality by each partner, and obviously no schizophrenia. Then there is multicellular parasitism, the extreme form being that of creatures living inside others (the unfortunate "hosts") where only the parasite benefits. Again, individuality is preserved—there are two or more independent Is (albeit the products of fusion) and no schizophrenia. And there are colonial multicellular forms (the coelonterata: medusae, jellyfish, hydrozoa) where creatures composed mainly of ectoderm and entoderm live as essentially radially symmetric forms with a central digestive tract and tentacles or tendrils which seize and immobilize prey and bring it to the mouth. In the hydrozoa, the principle structure may form buds that remain attached but survive independently if separated. Jellyfish may contain elements specialized to trap and immobilize prey, and other elements specialized in digestion. In case of separation, they survive independently—again, the colonial form is not schizophrenic. Therefore, healthy pluritissular organisms with multiple organs joined by peripheral nerve tracts to a central, coordinating nerve center (the brain) are not schizophrenic in normal circumstances. In humans, split-brain subjects do not become schizophrenic if they were not so before commissurotomy. Commissurotomy is the surgical transection of the corpus callosum, the principle commissure for information transfer between the cerebral hemispheres. The procedure has been used for intractable epilepsy where a focus of electrically abnormal discharges in one hemisphere "kindles" so-called "secondary foci" in the other. So long as these have not acquired autonomy, severing the corpus callosum may render the disease manageable with medications. The post-commissurotomy patient is a case of one hemisphere's not knowing what the other is doing, e.g. images in the right visual field (which are processed in the occipital lobe of the left hemisphere) can be named since the speech center is in the left hemisphere in 95% of right handers and 85-90% of left handers. Thus, a written word presented in the right visual field can be read aloud whereas it cannot be if presented in the left visual field, which is processed in the right occipital lobe. In partial complex epilepsy of the older "psychomotor" variety, victims appear to observers to carry out acts which seem purposeful but not goal-directed. There might be fiddling with clothes, apparently senseless repetitious movements or vocalizations, humming, attacks of rage and so on. Nonetheless, the patient progresses through the environment without suffering major injury. The "psychomotor" behavior(s) is/are inappropriate to the circumstances subjects are in, without aberrations of behavior sufficient to cause bodily harm to

the subject. In the form of e
motor seizures," conscious
retained and at others, lost.
retained, patients are aware of
body parts yet powerless to sto
seizures, a brain region conc
sensory modality is triggered b
foci rather than its peripheral
ple "see" flashing lights, "hea
"smell" and "taste" nonexis
stances, or "feel" contact on pa
istent) but know these to be
know this because the prepo
operating cerebral logic and a
clude that the false sensations
events at the body surface. The
preceding examples is, that
tions (by virtue of cerebral lo
cesses) and epileptic muscul
(bioelectrical) pathologies of
means that there is/are norma
lating the motor strip, while
the absence of triggered sens
mal stimulation of the recepto
bral(I) origin. The prerola
therefore a cortical receptor ar
sory receptor cortical areas, di
because the normal input to i
commanding muscular activit
matter/energy at the body surf
hallucinations requires that
"sensory" conclusions by fuse
rogue, or maverick, or malfun

phreni
interna
age or
at face
is emp
stinks
"I" i
tary m
experie
to mat
cellula
.That
skin. S
neural
one-ce
betwee
their n
sider it
the syn
macro
for the
If so
only l
other
zoans'
brane.
metazo
(sound
they in
inner e
ecules
to cul
engage

other hand, interpret only tactile sensation (skin contact) as "direct," and all other sensations as "long range." The physical reality is that all detections of macro matter/energy are made by organs at or recessed in the body surface, none remotely(!) near cerebral receptor neurons . Therefore all metazoan sensations are really long range, but because neural circuits , by a conceptual sleight of hand, render skin the equivalent of protozoan cell membranes, "touch sensation" is believed to be direct. Brains can survive loss of portions of the body surface if blood loss, shock and infection are controlled. Losing "my" hand, leg etc may be survivable precisely because non-neuronal cells, tissues and organs are not really the demarcation between brain cells and the non-brain macro world. But it is necessary for brains to believe this because the relative safety from microscopic dangers achieved with multicellular fortification of neurons obliges neural circuits to inventory and map out the macroscopic surface of the multicellular organism in order to appraise its macroscopic needs and dangers, and command displacements in the macro world. Accordingly, just as "sensations" must be elaborated de novo in each newborn multicellular being, so too must be elaborated, via a sequence of symbolic neural circuits and bioelectric processing, the concept of an animal's surface shape and dimensions. In fact, for logical reasons this necessarily must precede the elaboration of sensations. Sensations are discoverable and definable only by reference to the previously elaborated concept of the shape and dimensions of the cutaneous envelope. We have shown that they must be produced before a deadline age in early life. If deer and antelope require hours after birth to master standing which allows suckling, and days or weeks to master running; if human babies take weeks to master head control and turn in bed, months to sit and longer to crawl and stand, and one to two years to learn to walk, this must be because brains actively process variations of bioelectric potentials culminating in symbolic mapping of surface morphology, parts of which (limbs, tentacles, elephant trunks etc) can later be selectively mobilized. Also, surface dimensions become brains' units of measure or yardstick for measuring non-body micro items. The body surface symbolizes "I" and all else is "non-I."

ching the analytical process requires one
ement: a means of measurement, or compari-
bioelectric variations in two or more areas of
in. This means is a function of the reality that
l inputs and output are integrated (fused)
single, coherent whole. Since that whole
know it is composed of neural circuits in a
y compartmentalized brain, comparing varia-
sing spatial units is not possible for "I."
neural logic circuits can establish whether
ebral bioelectric variations occur simulta-
or not. Given a closed loop wherein cortical
netic neurons and cortical sensorimotor neu-
eflecting muscle activity at the body surface)
istered and found consistently and reproduc-
vary simultaneously or not, a scale of tempo-
ncies of skin areas from the brain (actually,
") can be formed. The shape and dimensions
are plotted in units of time (the relative laten-
muscle couples from "I" and between them-
[1] While it is the temporal distance of muscle
from "I" that is plotted, "I" equates muscles
erlying skin: when brains command limbs or
or ears to displace themselves, they are not
hat the cerebral command activates muscles
ing portions of skin. None of the reasoning
ing what varies, the need for loops between
and portions of the body surface, and the
available to brains to measure variations
rains, was possible before neurons were dis-
with silver stains in the 1890s. Added to pre-

igure 5 on page 53

Chapter 2: The Logically Necessary Sequence of Cognitive Development

All learning takes off from an arbitrary cognitive base. Elaboration of the concept of body surface shape and dimensions, which allows that of sensations, perceptions, ideas and Mind has got to be erected on a cognitive base laid by evolution and embryology. Through DNA, evolution determines the order of appearance of somatic sensori-motor tissues and organs, the brain and its compartmentalization, and peripheral and central nervous pathways linking sensory detectors with cortical receptor neurons and the cerebral motor strip with skeletal muscles. The motor strip is a receptor region whose neurons vary when receiving cerebrally-originating bioelectric potentials, unlike the sensory receptor neurons varying in response to potentials from the body surface. In humans, normal gestation is about nine months. By the sixth month, all tissues and organs as well as the brain and its neural connections from and to same, have formed. The fetus is in the overall "fetal flexion" posture with head flexed on trunk, thighs on hips, legs on thighs, feet on legs, arms on trunk and forearms on arms. It is inside the uterus, buffered from uterine walls and bony pelvis by amniotic fluid. Skeletal muscles have got to be relaying baseline, so-called "resting frequency" bioelectric potentials causing neurons to vary in a supplementary, sensorimotor cortical area—sensory, because eventually brains teach themselves to recognize when muscles contract and relax, and even to what degree. Sensorymotor, because the awareness concerns muscles and not skin. The primary "tactile" or skin sensory receptor ("somesthetic") cortical area is in the anterior parietal lobe behind the fissure of Rolando. As for the presumed supplementary sensorimotor strip, its hypothesized existence is justified by the fact that at some point of cognitive development we become able to determine and control the degrees of contraction and relaxation of paired (agonist-antagonist) skeletal muscles. This is why body builders can show off selected muscles, and some belly dancers move coins up and down their abdomens using only selected abdominal muscle groups. Inactive but not inert, fetal muscles transmit baseline-frequency potentials to the sensorimotor receptor cortex. Agonist-antagonist pairs vary inversely so that when one contracts the other relaxes (e.g. biceps and triceps brachii, or hamstrings and quadriceps in the thigh). It stands to reason that in the last trimester of pregnancy, brains create registries in the sensorimotor cortex reflecting inversely varying agonist-antagonist muscle pairs, although the meaning of the registered phenomena remains to be discovered because other cerebral neuronal variations beginning at birth are needed to solve the puzzle. The forming of intracerebral registries occurs sans conscious deliberation. It is a consequence of obligatory cerebral reception of bioelectric potentials from triggered somatic sensors. For practical purposes, all sensors except those concerned with muscular contraction/relaxation, become active in a statistically significant way at birth and not in utero. Of course, the fact that

variations concern cerebral cel
ity, and heads is never factored
cess. In utero, environmental
energy, molecules triggering t
cells cannot be stimulating sen
ckel's discs, Paccinian corpuscl
cells, retinal rod and cone cel
starting at birth, the brain is
time by bioelectric potentials fr
sors , most significantly from t
by contact with non-body, non
only data "bank" brains have
of the new variations (althoug
data is to be found in the pro
new intracerebral variations
inversely varying skeletal r
although all cerebral sensory r
varying at birth, only variation
rons allow elaboration of a f
("tact"), whose discovery by
involves the sensorimotor (mu
rating the remaining sensory
must await the neural disco
since all learning builds on a
ceptual (data) foundations, the
the inverse agonist-antagonist
vides the concrete detail permi
logical/data-averaging symboli
of "somesthetic" cerebral rec
nating in discovery and neural
sation," "tact," followed by dis
of a species' other sense modal

Laur
other e
son, of
the bra
cerebr
into a
doesn'
spatial
tions
Rather
intrace
neousl
somest
rons (
are reg
ibly to
ral lat
from "
of skin
cies of
selves
couple
with o
trunks
aware
underl
concer
brains
option
inside
covere

1. See

vious discoveries (of bioelectricity, gross cerebral anatomy and compartmentalization, and links of "sense organs" to specific cerebral compartments), the discovery of neurons finally made clear that Mind is just as material as body, but in a different way. The Cartesian hypothesis of a mind-body duality could be refuted. It remains, "only," to show how neurons constitute Mind. The demonstration involves what we are doing: reasoning out how symbolic structural/dynamic variations of neural circuits and bioelectricity process intracerebral bioelectric variations culminating in symbolic neural/bioelectric concepts of body surface morphology and non-body items. All hierarchical levels of consciousness are symbolic conclusions (end products) of awareness-producing "machines" called neural circuits, which process bioelectric potentials. All brains are self-programmed to produce cognition, and all brains begin "production" when cerebral receptor neurons begin varying in electrical state in response to signals from somatic sensory detectors starting at birth. The only material resource available to neurons (which don't know they are that) to compare intracerebral bioelectric variations (which they are unaware of) is other neurons. The comparisons (or measurements) are performed never knowing that they concern variations separated by cerebral space, transmitted from and to non-nervous tissues far from brains (which they are unaware of) along tracts composed of nerve cells (both peripheral and cerebral). The only comparative modality possible in these circumstances is simultaneity, or non-simultaneity of variations in time. This is a binary logical invariable. In essence, all hierarchical stages of symbolic cerebral neural processing necessarily involve binary logic. If particular variations are invariable, consistent and reproducible by "I," then a particular, arbitrary and idiosyncratic form of time (distance in temporal latencies of skeletal muscle couples from "I") becomes I's only means of measuring distances of muscles from itself and relative to each other. "I" does not know the measured variables are muscles—when we command hands to grasp or toes to curl we believe the commands go to the anatomic structures, hands/feet, demarcated from non-I by skin. That is, we believe we are mobilizing skin and its content, not muscles. Once acquired, this concept of time, arbitrary and idiosyncratic, enables "I" to map (thereby defining) the shape, proportions and dimensions of the body surface which becomes "I" to the fused cerebral inputs/output that are the real "I." The symbolic intracerebral product of integrated inputs/output, unaware that that is what it is, assigns identity of the multicellular collective it manages (whose histology it is unaware of) to that portion it discovered in an ascending cascade of binary, symbolic logical and data-averaging steps: the skin, considered the boundary between self and non-self.

Delivery from wombs or eggs passively reverses the flexed posture of fetuses. The baby is mechanically straightened by its passage through the bony pelvic opening or the opening in egg shells. Flexor muscles are passively elongated while antagonist extensors passively shorten. This causes variation in the inversely varying muscle couples. The variation direct routes so as to minimize synaptic snarls nags.

ce learning builds upon prior cognitive bases, ature of macroscopic long-range sensations has discovered in function of a first-elaborated, and ed, macroscopic direct sensation. That is what xperience as "tact:" awareness of the corporal ope and items juxtaposed to it. Its elaboration res consistent, reproducible intracortical neural tions ("I" can register the variations, but not they are neural). The only variations fitting criteria are the feedback (sensorimotor) nses of skeletal muscles ordered to vary by "I" h considers it is mobilizing segments of the surface as it knows nothing of muscles) and ack responses of areas of skin to the somatosen- cortex when commands to parts of "the body" ally, to selected muscles) bring body parts into ct. Babies must learn each of these things: first, nmand specific muscles ("body parts"), then to une the excursions of limb segments in space so appose two body segments to each other. Ath- musicians, acrobats, yogis and others spend all lives refining these two forms of control. Much ants' growth is devoted to mastering skeletal les. Life outside the womb begins with little or uscle control. That is acquired in stages. Even- , mastery may develop beyond that necessary ocomotion and basic dexterity. Examples in ns have been given. Animals may be taught tural skills: riding bicycles (also unnatural for ns), bipedal walking (circus dogs and felines), ng with balls (seals) etc. The physical circuits

is relayed to sensorimotor receptor neurons in the brain. For the first time, the symbolic and as-yet unidentified flexor/extensor muscles registry elaborated in the last trimester of gestation, varies in a statistically quantitative significant degree. Soon, also for the first time, baby's skin contacts rigid non-body, non-amniotic matter. Gravity ensures that some segment of skin always contact non-body matter. Aquatic creatures must, for the first time, push the entire integument against salt or fresh water. Cutaneous detectors of matter/energy such as Paccinian corpuscles and Merckel's discs are triggered. Bioelectric potentials are relayed to the "somatosensory" or "somesthetic" cortices (one in each cerebral hemisphere). In humans, this is located in the anterior parietal lobe, behind the fissure of Rolando. Anterior to the fissure is the motor strip. I have argued that the motor strip (not to be confused with the sensorimotor strip which receives signals from skeletal muscle couples undergoing inverse variations in electrical state) is a receptor cortex—it receives commands of cerebral origin ("I") to vary contractions/relaxations of specific muscle couples. The somatosensory and motor strips, and doubtless their supplementary areas are the only receptor cortices with a homuncular topography. Homunculi are caricatural humans (or, in monkey brains, caricatural monkeys) arched backwards over the fissure of Rolando, feet in the mesial (interhemispheric) portion of the hemisphere at the bottom, leg and thigh vertically above, pelvis-abdomen-torso spilling over the top, and shoulder, arm, forearm and hand in the superior to inferior convexity. The hand is at the bottom of the convexity in front of the face. The thumb is disproportionately large, as are the lips (ergo, caricature). The sensory homunculus (one per hemisphere) is plotted by stimulating portions of skin and recording with electrodes where, in the somatosensory strip, the signal arrives. Signals from a same portion of skin always activate neurons in the same part of the strip. The motor homunculus is plotted by stimulating localized portions of the motor strip and noting which muscles respond at the body surface. The same portion of strip always activates the same muscles. There is no homunculus in the visual, olfactory, auditory and gustatory receptor regions. This is because there is a cortical— cutaneous sensors—cortical and a cortical—skeletal muscles—cortical feedback loop whose activation and logical analysis within brains enables them to elaborate tactile sensation and plot the surface envelope of the body. There are no cortical—peripheral organ—cortical loops for long-range macroscopic senses. A closed loop system of two functionally related variables ("tactile" and muscular "sensations") is mathematically indispensable to discover the significance of each from inside the head. Logical-symbolic processing of intracortical bioelectric variations necessitates material (synaptic) links between homologous sections of the motor and somesthetic strips and probably also supplementary receptor strips. The homuncular topography minimizes risks of synaptic snags and snarls and is therefore an embodiement of bioelectric wiring efficiency.

Cerebral neurons are unaware of themselves and of being in brains contained in heads which, in turn,

form part of a multicellular organis
ural selection, evolution has fashion
logic and topographic juxtaposition
programmed elaboration of cons
macroscopic. For logical reasons,
orders of sentience: sensations, p
must be constructed by neuronal ci
sequence. The building blocks on w
edifice rests are somatosensation
sensation. Now, a single neuron o
nected neurons alone, are insuff
variations of cortical sensory rece
minating in symbolic conclusions t
body envelope, a non-body world b
ple non-body phenomena in the
pressures, textures, temperature
odors and flavors etc. Structurally,
cally logical device enabling cerebr
cover the macro being they m
physical items external to it, is t
neurons to form cell circuits for sy
intracortical bioelectric variations.
cessing is binary. The primordial
involves variation or not of (sensc
rons. What "I" must process is w
have or have not occurred. It never
varies is neurons. There must be
lytical cascade, from simplest to
consecutive cell circuits functionin
(Boolean or other) to culminate in
cognitive sophistication. Bioelec
increasingly complex cell circuits
coherent input-output whole, {I}),

and specific neural variations serving as points of departure for acquiring muscle control are arbitrary and the products of evolution and embryology: physical pathways linking stimulated skin sensors to the somatosensory cortex; segmental (spinal cord and motor nerve) pathways producing reflex variations of flexor/extensor muscle couples under areas of stimulated skin {the polysynaptic reflex}; pathways linking muscles with the sensorimotor cortex (for relaying signals concerning muscle couple variations; and, pathways from the cortical motor strip (controlled by "I") to specific muscles. Brains learn to activate muscles after registering muscle variations caused by the above-mentioned polysynaptic reflex. A description of same may be found in all basic neurophysiology books. At this point ,brains — recognizing that signals arrive when "I" has stimulated body parts (muscles) but also when "I" has not {reflex variations}) — must logically deduce that said variations may be induced either by "I" or "non-I." Therefore, there is a non-I world.

Reflexes are stereotyped muscle responses to local stimuli. In the Babinski reflex, stimuli to the sole of the foot cause extension of the big toe followed by extension and fanning of the other toes. It becomes inhibited at about eighteen months of age, reappearing in pathological circumstances. In the triple-retreat reflex, stimulating any part of the lower extremity causes flexion of foot on leg, leg on thigh and thigh on hip. In the upper extremities, stimulating the palm causes extension of hand on forearm, forearm on arm, and abduction of arm from shoulder. Now, the idea, "equality," involves linkage. Physically, that which links two or more constants/ variables declared equal is a matter of convention. As we have argued often before, central nervous system options for physical links joining equal factors are materially few—in fact, only synaptic links may constitute equal signs (or associations which do not signify equality). Therefore, structural/dynamic foci of bioelectricity representing symbolic conclusions of processed variations of bioelectricity performed by successive neural circuits, and separate in cerebral space, are either "equal," or associated but not equal, when linked synaptically. Synapses are bioelectric junctions of upstream-downstream neurons. Neurons consist of a cell body containing the nucleus, dendrites which are filaments connecting with downstream cells, and axons which are filaments connecting with upstream cells. Dendrite-axon junctions are called synaptic clefts. Cerebral neurons are either excitatory (Golgi type I cell) or inhibitory (Golgi type II). The former activate downstream neurons causing bioelectric variation, by emitting chemicals such as acetylcholine ("AcChol"). The latter inhibit activation of downstream neurons with chemicals such as gammaaminobutyric acid ("GABA"). Bioelectric variations of the cell body are caused by exchanges of sodium and potassium across the cell membrane, and also magnesium. Some excess ions and chemical mediators (e.g. GABA and AcChol) are disposed of by white brain cells called glia (so-called "sink action"). Glia also play an immunologic role, which doesn't concern us, and are important for synapse formation (according to recent publications) which concerns us greatly.

It is estimated that the average human brain contains about one hundred billion neurons (gray cells). Another estimate is that a neuron may synapse with about one thousand others[2]. "The brain has about a hundred million neurons, each connected to about a thousand other cells; simply producing any sort of a wiring diagram is a monumental project."

View these numbers, the possibilities of synaptic misdirection appear astronomical. Evolution and embryology produced the somatosensory and sensori-motor homunculi precisely to minimize synaptic glitches. Exposure of babies to all sensory stimuli from birth, and the presence of the polysynaptic reflex arc, allows cell circuits downstream of the sensorimotor and somatosensory homunculi to discover that there is a body envelope by elaborating the sensation called "tact" or "somesthesia." No pathways nor reflexes permit direct cerebral discovery and therefore definition of the macroscopic long-range sensations. The concepts, "tact" and "body surface" are the foundation for elaborating sight, hearing, olfaction and gustation in humans, and other sensations in non-humans such as echolocation or long range detection of bioelectricity. Suppose there were no somesthetic nor sensorimotor homunculi and stimulation of the same area of skin always caused cerebral neurons to vary in random, never-the-same parts of the cortex. And cerebral cortical orders to specific muscles always departed from random, never -the-same cortical regions; or, signals from the

2. David C. Noelle, "Exorcising The Homunculus" in "free inquiry," Spring 2001, VOL21 No.2, p.32.

same skin area always arrived in the same cortical locus but these loci were not grouped in a single cortical strip but mixed helter-skelter with some signals from green-detecting retinal cells, and neurons ordering contraction of a shoulder muscle, neurons activated by cochlear cells detecting sound in the 2000—3000 Hz frequency, and yet others controlling eye movements. Establishing synaptic equal signs between homologous cerebral areas receiving signals from the skin of the right thumb and neurons controlling underlying muscles is impossible. Yet such links must form for brains (actually, their "Is") to discover that variations concerning stimulated thumb skin are topographically related to cerebral variations commanding underlying muscles—which "I" believes are the thumb. Suppose that signals to and from cerebral neurons always varied in the same cerebral locus, but those from left thumb adjoined those from the red band of the visible spectrum, etc. Here, the likelihood of synaptic snags and glitches is very high It follows that the sensorimotor and somatosensory homunculi are not intracerebral little men observing themselves, but cases of optimal synaptic wiring minimizing the risk of misdirected linking.

Chapter 3: The Mechanics, Symbolism and Sequence of Cognitive Elaboration

Neural circuits are the only material resource brains have for processing bioelectric potentials of extracerebral origin so as to elaborate consciousness. Because they both produce and form the hierarchical orders of awareness (sensations, perceptions, ideas),the geometry of cell circuits, and bioelectric variations in and between them must be symbolically meaningful. Circuits are needed because single cells cannot symbolically build nor stand for concepts (awareness). At most, single neurons may function as "AND" gates in a Boolean or some other symbolic logic system. That is because through synaptic connections with downstream neurons, they may be excited to vary, or not. Basic histology teaches that neurons are triggered (vary) by spatial or temporal stimulation, or both. Through their synapses with downstream neurons, activation may occur if a critical number of potentials arrives simultaneously (causing the cell body to discharge bioelectricity), or discharge may require trains of incoming potentials sufficiently close in time. Or, both mechanisms may be needed. But an AND gate in isolation is symbolically insufficient for performing logical analysis leading to conclusions. Also needed are NOT and OR gates. These can be formed only by particular circuit geometries (ergo multiple neurons) as we show later.

The human neocortex has six layers, each subdivided in smaller layers. Neurons are disposed vertically and horizontally in and between layers. Excitatory and inhibitory neurons are either at rest electrically, or active. When a cell, or several in a circuit, vary or not, we have the symbolic equivalent of binary 1s and 0s. Horizontal and vertical layering, and neural connections in and between cortical cell layers, could represent circuits processing bioelectric variations in increasingly complex order

For cell circuits to conclude that variations are signals from a body envelope (i.e. that there exists a body surface), they must compare variations in time (whether simultaneous or not). To do this, they must have immediate memory. It was argued before that "I" cannot compare variations in cerebral space—it doesn't know it is a fusion of neuronal bioelectric inputs and outputs contained in something called "brain." Let memory be defined as the physical persistence of a bioelectric neural variation be it of one cell or a cell-circuit, when the varying cell or circuit has varied yet again. The only intracerebral matter available to satisfy this definition is neurons upstream of the varying cell or circuit, linked to same and disposed in space so as to retain the variation when the downstream phenomenon varies yet again. Accordingly, the first tier of neurons varying in response to peripheral signals, must be linked to upstream tiers in such manner that to a third, or monitoring tier, some neurons of the second tier correspond to the prevarying first-tier neurons, and others to the varying neurons. Upstream logic cirthis generation is professor Lynn Margulis. Said hypothesis affirms that some intracellular inclusions in eukaryotes were originally independent microorganisms (ribosomes, mitochondria, endoplasmic reticulum). There was presumably a first stage of symbiosis, and over geologic time spans symbiosis led to fusion, resulting in single-celled biota of some internal complexity. At the multicellular scale, there are clearly cases of symbiosis (e.g. fish living between the tentacles of sea anemones, luring others to the tentacles and feeding on scraps). There is a mutually beneficial relationship with retention of individuality by each partner, and obviously no schizophrenia. Then there is multicellular parasitism, the extreme form being that of creatures living inside others (the unfortunate "hosts") where only the parasite benefits. Again, individuality is preserved—there are two or more independent Is (albeit the products of fusion) and no schizophrenia. And there are colonial multicellular forms (the coelonterata: medusae, jellyfish, hydrozoa) where creatures composed mainly of ectoderm and entoderm live as essentially radially symmetric forms with a central digestive tract and tentacles or tendrils which seize and immobilize prey and bring it to the mouth. In the hydrozoa, the principle structure may form buds that remain attached but survive independently if separated. Jellyfish may contain elements specialized to trap and immobilize prey, and other elements specialized in digestion. In case of separation, they survive independently—again, the colonial form is not schizophrenic. Therefore, healthy pluritissular organisms with multiple organs joined by peripheral nerve tracts to a central, coordinating nerve center (the brain) are not schizophrenic in normal circumstances. In humans, split-brain subjects do not become schizophrenic if they were not so before commissurotomy. Commissurotomy is the surgical transection of the corpus callosum, the principle commissure for information transfer between the cerebral hemispheres. The procedure has been used for intractable epilepsy where a focus of electrically abnormal discharges in one hemisphere "kindles" so-called "secondary foci" in the other. So long as these have not acquired autonomy, severing the corpus callosum may render the disease manageable with medications. The post-commissurotomy patient is a case of one hemisphere's not knowing what the other is doing, e.g. images in the right visual field (which are processed in the occipital lobe of the left hemisphere) can be named since the speech center is in the left hemisphere in 95% of right handers and 85-90% of left handers. Thus, a written word presented in the right visual field can be read aloud whereas it cannot be if presented in the left visual field, which is processed in the right occipital lobe. In partial complex epilepsy of the older "psychomotor" variety, victims appear to observers to carry out acts which seem purposeful but not goal-directed. There might be fiddling with clothes, apparently senseless repetitious movements or vocalizations, humming, attacks of rage and so on. Nonetheless, the patient progresses through the environment without suffering major injury. The "psychomotor" behavior(s) is/are inappropriate to the circumstances subjects are in, without aberrations of behavior sufficient to cause bodily harm to

Chapter 2: The Logically Necessary Sequence of Cognitive Development

All learning takes off from an arbitrary cognitive base. Elaboration of the concept of body surface shape and dimensions, which allows that of sensations, perceptions, ideas and Mind has got to be erected on a cognitive base laid by evolution and embryology. Through DNA, evolution determines the order of appearance of somatic sensori-motor tissues and organs, the brain and its compartmentalization, and peripheral and central nervous pathways linking sensory detectors with cortical receptor neurons and the cerebral motor strip with skeletal muscles. The motor strip is a receptor region whose neurons vary when receiving cerebrally-originating bioelectric potentials, unlike the sensory receptor neurons varying in response to potentials from the body surface. In humans, normal gestation is about nine months. By the sixth month, all tissues and organs as well as the brain and its neural connections from and to same, have formed. The fetus is in the overall "fetal flexion" posture with head flexed on trunk, thighs on hips, legs on thighs, feet on legs, arms on trunk and forearms on arms. It is inside the uterus, buffered from uterine walls and bony pelvis by amniotic fluid. Skeletal muscles have got to be relaying baseline, so-called "resting frequency" bioelectric potentials causing neurons to vary in a supplementary, sensorimotor cortical area—sensory, because eventually brains teach themselves to recognize when muscles contract and relax, and even to what degree. Sensorymotor, because the awareness concerns muscles and not skin. The primary "tactile" or skin sensory receptor ("somesthetic") cortical area is in the anterior parietal lobe behind the fissure of Rolando. As for the presumed supplementary sensorimotor strip, its hypothesized existence is justified by the fact that at some point of cognitive development we become able to determine and control the degrees of contraction and relaxation of paired (agonist-antagonist) skeletal muscles. This is why body builders can show off selected muscles, and some belly dancers move coins up and down their abdomens using only selected abdominal muscle groups. Inactive but not inert, fetal muscles transmit baseline-frequency potentials to the sensorimotor receptor cortex. Agonist-antagonist pairs vary inversely so that when one contracts the other relaxes (e.g. biceps and triceps brachii, or hamstrings and quadriceps in the thigh). It stands to reason that in the last trimester of pregnancy, brains create registries in the sensorimotor cortex reflecting inversely varying agonist-antagonist muscle pairs, although the meaning of the registered phenomena remains to be discovered because other cerebral neuronal variations beginning at birth are needed to solve the puzzle. The forming of intracerebral registries occurs sans conscious deliberation. It is a consequence of obligatory cerebral reception of bioelectric potentials from triggered somatic sensors. For practical purposes, all sensors except those concerned with muscular contraction/relaxation, become active in a statistically significant way at birth and not in utero. Of course, the fact that vious discoveries (of bioelectricity, gross cerebral anatomy and compartmentalization, and links of "sense organs" to specific cerebral compartments), the discovery of neurons finally made clear that Mind is just as material as body, but in a different way. The Cartesian hypothesis of a mind-body duality could be refuted. It remains, "only," to show how neurons constitute Mind. The demonstration involves what we are doing: reasoning out how symbolic structural/dynamic variations of neural circuits and bioelectricity process intracerebral bioelectric variations culminating in symbolic neural/bioelectric concepts of body surface morphology and non-body items. All hierarchical levels of consciousness are symbolic conclusions (end products) of awareness-producing "machines" called neural circuits, which process bioelectric potentials. All brains are self-programmed to produce cognition, and all brains begin "production" when cerebral receptor neurons begin varying in electrical state in response to signals from somatic sensory detectors starting at birth. The only material resource available to neurons (which don't know they are that) to compare intracerebral bioelectric variations (which they are unaware of) is other neurons. The comparisons (or measurements) are performed never knowing that they concern variations separated by cerebral space, transmitted from and to non-nervous tissues far from brains (which they are unaware of) along tracts composed of nerve cells (both peripheral and cerebral). The only comparative modality possible in these circumstances is simultaneity, or non-simultaneity of variations in time. This is a binary logical invariable. In essence, all hierarchical stages of symbolic cerebral neural processing necessarily involve binary logic. If particular variations are invariable, consistent and reproducible by "I," then a particular, arbitrary and idiosyncratic form of time (distance in temporal latencies of skeletal muscle couples from "I") becomes I's only means of measuring distances of muscles from itself and relative to each other. "I" does not know the measured variables are muscles—when we command hands to grasp or toes to curl we believe the commands go to the anatomic structures, hands/feet, demarcated from non-I by skin. That is, we believe we are mobilizing skin and its content, not muscles. Once acquired, this concept of time, arbitrary and idiosyncratic, enables "I" to map (thereby defining) the shape, proportions and dimensions of the body surface which becomes "I" to the fused cerebral inputs/output that are the real "I." The symbolic intracerebral product of integrated inputs/output, unaware that that is what it is, assigns identity of the multicellular collective it manages (whose histology it is unaware of) to that portion it discovered in an ascending cascade of binary, symbolic logical and data-averaging steps: the skin, considered the boundary between self and non-self.

Delivery from wombs or eggs passively reverses the flexed posture of fetuses. The baby is mechanically straightened by its passage through the bony pelvic opening or the opening in egg shells. Flexor muscles are passively elongated while antagonist extensors passively shorten. This causes variation in the inversely varying muscle couples. The variation is relayed to sensorimotor receptor neurons in the brain. For the first time, the symbolic and as-yet unidentified flexor/extensor muscles registry elaborated in the last trimester of gestation, varies in a statistically quantitative significant degree. Soon, also for the first time, baby's skin contacts rigid non-body, non-amniotic matter. Gravity ensures that some segment of skin always contact non-body matter. Aquatic creatures must, for the first time, push the entire integument against salt or fresh water. Cutaneous detectors of matter/energy such as Paccinian corpuscles and Merckel's discs are triggered. Bioelectric potentials are relayed to the "somatosensory" or "somesthetic" cortices (one in each cerebral hemisphere). In humans, this is located in the anterior parietal lobe, behind the fissure of Rolando. Anterior to the fissure is the motor strip. I have argued that the motor strip (not to be confused with the sensorimotor strip which receives signals from skeletal muscle couples undergoing inverse variations in electrical state) is a receptor cortex—it receives commands of cerebral origin ("I") to vary contractions/relaxations of specific muscle couples. The somatosensory and motor strips, and doubtless their supplementary areas are the only receptor cortices with a homuncular topography. Homunculi are caricatural humans (or, in monkey brains, caricatural monkeys) arched backwards over the fissure of Rolando, feet in the mesial (interhemispheric) portion of the hemisphere at the bottom, leg and thigh vertically above, pelvis-abdomen-torso spilling over the top, and shoulder, arm, forearm and hand in the superior to inferior convexity. The hand is at the bottom of the convexity in front of the face. The thumb is disproportionately large, as are the lips (ergo, caricature). The sensory homunculus (one per hemisphere) is plotted by stimulating portions of skin and recording with electrodes where, in the somatosensory strip, the signal arrives. Signals from a same portion of skin always activate neurons in the same part of the strip. The motor homunculus is plotted by stimulating localized portions of the motor strip and noting which muscles respond at the body surface. The same portion of strip always activates the same muscles. There is no homunculus in the visual, olfactory, auditory and gustatory receptor regions. This is because there is a cortical— cutaneous sensors—cortical and a cortical—skeletal muscles—cortical feedback loop whose activation and logical analysis within brains enables them to elaborate tactile sensation and plot the surface envelope of the body. There are no cortical—peripheral organ—cortical loops for long-range macroscopic senses. A closed loop system of two functionally related variables ("tactile" and muscular "sensations") is mathematically indispensable to discover the significance of each from inside the head. Logical-symbolic processing of intracortical bioelectric variations necessitates material (synaptic) links between homologous sections of the motor and somesthetic strips and probably also supplementary receptor strips. The homuncular topography minimizes risks of synaptic snags and snarls and is therefore an embodiement of bioelectric wiring efficiency.

Cerebral neurons are unaware of themselves and of being in brains contained in heads which, in turn, and specific neural variations serving as points of departure for acquiring muscle control are arbitrary and the products of evolution and embryology: physical pathways linking stimulated skin sensors to the somatosensory cortex; segmental (spinal cord and motor nerve) pathways producing reflex variations of flexor/extensor muscle couples under areas of stimulated skin {the polysynaptic reflex}; pathways linking muscles with the sensorimotor cortex (for relaying signals concerning muscle couple variations; and, pathways from the cortical motor strip (controlled by "I") to specific muscles. Brains learn to activate muscles after registering muscle variations caused by the above-mentioned polysynaptic reflex. A description of same may be found in all basic neurophysiology books. At this point ,brains — recognizing that signals arrive when "I" has stimulated body parts (muscles) but also when "I" has not {reflex variations}) — must logically deduce that said variations may be induced either by "I" or "non-I." Therefore, there is a non-I world.

Reflexes are stereotyped muscle responses to local stimuli. In the Babinski reflex, stimuli to the sole of the foot cause extension of the big toe followed by extension and fanning of the other toes. It becomes inhibited at about eighteen months of age, reappearing in pathological circumstances. In the triple-retreat reflex, stimulating any part of the lower extremity causes flexion of foot on leg, leg on thigh and thigh on hip. In the upper extremities, stimulating the palm causes extension of hand on forearm, forearm on arm, and abduction of arm from shoulder. Now, the idea, "equality," involves linkage. Physically, that which links two or more constants/variables declared equal is a matter of convention. As we have argued often before, central nervous system options for physical links joining equal factors are materially few—in fact, only synaptic links may constitute equal signs (or associations which do not signify equality). Therefore, structural/dynamic foci of bioelectricity representing symbolic conclusions of processed variations of bioelectricity performed by successive neural circuits, and separate in cerebral space, are either "equal," or associated but not equal, when linked synaptically. Synapses are bioelectric junctions of upstream-downstream neurons. Neurons consist of a cell body containing the nucleus, dendrites which are filaments connecting with downstream cells, and axons which are filaments connecting with upstream cells. Dendrite-axon junctions are called synaptic clefts. Cerebral neurons are either excitatory (Golgi type I cell) or inhibitory (Golgi type II). The former activate downstream neurons causing bioelectric variation, by emitting chemicals such as acetylcholine ("AcChol"). The latter inhibit activation of downstream neurons with chemicals such as gammaaminobutyric acid ("GABA"). Bioelectric variations of the cell body are caused by exchanges of sodium and potassium across the cell membrane, and also magnesium. Some excess ions and chemical mediators (e.g. GABA and AcChol) are disposed of by white brain cells called glia (so-called "sink action"). Glia also play an immunologic role, which doesn't concern us, and are important for synapse formation (according to recent publications) which concerns us greatly.

form part of a multicellular organism. Through natural selection, evolution has fashioned optimal histologic and topographic juxtapositions permitting self-programmed elaboration of consciousness of the macroscopic. For logical reasons, the hierarchical orders of sentience: sensations, perceptions, ideas, must be constructed by neuronal circuits in a logical sequence. The building blocks on which the cognitive edifice rests are somatosensation and sensorimotor sensation. Now, a single neuron or a few interconnected neurons alone, are insufficient to process variations of cortical sensory receptor neurons culminating in symbolic conclusions that there exists a body envelope, a non-body world beyond, and multiple non-body phenomena in the non-body realm: pressures, textures, temperatures, sound, light, odors and flavors etc. Structurally, the only symbolically logical device enabling cerebral neurons to discover the macro being they must control, and physical items external to it, is the connection of neurons to form cell circuits for symbolic parsing of intracortical bioelectric variations. All symbolic processing is binary. The primordial binary processing involves variation or not of (sensory receptor) neurons. What "I" must process is whether variations have or have not occurred. It never knows that what varies is neurons. There must be an ascending analytical cascade, from simplest to most complex, via consecutive cell circuits functioning in a logic system (Boolean or other) to culminate in lesser or greater cognitive sophistication. Bioelectricity in these increasingly complex cell circuits (fused into one coherent input-output whole, {I}), should follow the most direct routes so as to minimize synaptic snarls and snags.

Since learning builds upon prior cognitive bases, the nature of macroscopic long-range sensations has to be discovered in function of a first-elaborated, and defined, macroscopic direct sensation. That is what we experience as "tact:" awareness of the corporal envelope and items juxtaposed to it. Its elaboration requires consistent, reproducible intracortical neural variations ("I" can register the variations, but not that they are neural). The only variations fitting these criteria are the feedback (sensorimotor) responses of skeletal muscles ordered to vary by "I" (which considers it is mobilizing segments of the body surface as it knows nothing of muscles) and feedback responses of areas of skin to the somatosensory cortex when commands to parts of "the body" (actually, to selected muscles) bring body parts into contact. Babies must learn each of these things: first, to command specific muscles ("body parts"), then to fine-tune the excursions of limb segments in space so as to appose two body segments to each other. Athletes, musicians, acrobats, yogis and others spend all their lives refining these two forms of control. Much of infants' growth is devoted to mastering skeletal muscles. Life outside the womb begins with little or no muscle control. That is acquired in stages. Eventually, mastery may develop beyond that necessary for locomotion and basic dexterity. Examples in humans have been given. Animals may be taught unnatural skills: riding bicycles (also unnatural for humans), bipedal walking (circus dogs and felines), playing with balls (seals) etc. The physical circuits variations concern cerebral cells, brains, bioelectricity, and heads is never factored in the analytical process. In utero, environmental light, sound, matter/energy, molecules triggering taste buds and nasal cells cannot be stimulating sensors in the skin (Merckel's discs, Paccinian corpuscles et al), cochlear hair cells, retinal rod and cone cells etc. It follows that starting at birth, the brain is deluged for the first time by bioelectric potentials from all peripheral sensors , most significantly from those in skin triggered by contact with non-body, non-amniotic items. The only data "bank" brains have to start making sense of the new variations (although the meaning of said data is to be found in the process of analyzing the new intracerebral variations) is the registry of inversely varying skeletal muscle couples. And although all cerebral sensory receptor neurons begin varying at birth, only variations of somesthetic neurons allow elaboration of a first sensory modality ("tact"), whose discovery by the brain necessarily involves the sensorimotor (muscles) registry. Elaborating the remaining sensory modalities of a species must await the neural discovery of "tact." Thus, since all learning builds on arbitrary, previous conceptual (data) foundations, the in utero formation of the inverse agonist-antagonist muscles registry provides the concrete detail permitting the launching of logical/data-averaging symbolic analysis of variations of "somesthetic" cerebral receptor neurons culminating in discovery and neural definition of the "sensation," "tact," followed by discovery and definitions of a species' other sense modalities.

Launching the analytical process requires one other element: a means of measurement, or comparison, of bioelectric variations in two or more areas of the brain. This means is a function of the reality that cerebral inputs and output are integrated (fused) into a single, coherent whole. Since that whole doesn't know it is composed of neural circuits in a spatially compartmentalized brain, comparing variations using spatial units is not possible for "I." Rather, neural logic circuits can establish whether intracerebral bioelectric variations occur simultaneously or not. Given a closed loop wherein cortical somesthetic neurons and cortical sensorimotor neurons (reflecting muscle activity at the body surface) are registered and found consistently and reproducibly to vary simultaneously or not, a scale of temporal latencies of skin areas from the brain (actually, from "I") can be formed. The shape and dimensions of skin are plotted in units of time (the relative latencies of muscle couples from "I" and between themselves).[1] While it is the temporal distance of muscle couples from "I" that is plotted, "I" equates muscles with overlying skin: when brains command limbs or trunks or ears to displace themselves, they are not aware that the cerebral command activates muscles underlying portions of skin. None of the reasoning concerning what varies, the need for loops between brains and portions of the body surface, and the options available to brains to measure variations inside brains, was possible before neurons were discovered with silver stains in the 1890s. Added to pre-

---

1. See Figure 5 on page 53

deadline age in early life. If deer and antelope require hours after birth to master standing which allows suckling, and days or weeks to master running; if human babies take weeks to master head control and turn in bed, months to sit and longer to crawl and stand, and one to two years to learn to walk, this must be because brains actively process variations of bioelectric potentials culminating in symbolic mapping of surface morphology, parts of which (limbs, tentacles, elephant trunks etc) can later be selectively mobilized. Also, surface dimensions become brains' units of measure or yardstick for measuring non-body micro items. The body surface symbolizes "I" and all else is "non-I."

other hand, interpret only tactile sensation (skin contact) as "direct," and all other sensations as "long range." The physical reality is that all detections of macro matter/energy are made by organs at or recessed in the body surface, none remotely(!) near cerebral receptor neurons . Therefore all metazoan sensations are really long range, but because neural circuits , by a conceptual sleight of hand, render skin the equivalent of protozoan cell membranes, "touch sensation" is believed to be direct. Brains can survive loss of portions of the body surface if blood loss, shock and infection are controlled. Losing "my" hand, leg etc may be survivable precisely because non-neuronal cells, tissues and organs are not really the demarcation between brain cells and the non-brain macro world. But it is necessary for brains to believe this because the relative safety from microscopic dangers achieved with multicellular fortification of neurons obliges neural circuits to inventory and map out the macroscopic surface of the multicellular organism in order to appraise its macroscopic needs and dangers, and command displacements in the macro world. Accordingly, just as "sensations" must be elaborated de novo in each newborn multicellular being, so too must be elaborated, via a sequence of symbolic neural circuits and bioelectric processing, the concept of an animal's surface shape and dimensions. In fact, for logical reasons this necessarily must precede the elaboration of sensations. Sensations are discoverable and definable only by reference to the previously elaborated concept of the shape and dimensions of the cutaneous envelope. We have shown that they must be produced before a the subject. In the form of epilepsy called "major motor seizures," consciousness is sometimes retained and at others, lost. In cases where it is retained, patients are aware of tonic-clonic jerking of body parts yet powerless to stop it. In purely sensory seizures, a brain region concerned with a specific sensory modality is triggered by pathologic cerebral foci rather than its peripheral sensory detector. People "see" flashing lights, "hear" inarticulate voices, "smell" and "taste" nonexistent odors and substances, or "feel" contact on parts of the skin (nonexistent) but know these to be hallucinations. They know this because the preponderance of normally operating cerebral logic and averaging circuits conclude that the false sensations are not supported by events at the body surface. The significance of all the preceding examples is, that recognizing hallucinations (by virtue of cerebral logic and averaging processes) and epileptic muscular contractions to be (bioelectrical) pathologies of (local) areas of "I" means that there is/are normal (cerebral) foci stimulating the motor strip, while sensory experiences in the absence of triggered sense organs imply abnormal stimulation of the receptor cortices of local cerebral(I) origin. The prerolandic motor strip is therefore a cortical receptor area like the sundry sensory receptor cortical areas, differing from them only because the normal input to it is a cerebral one ("I" commanding muscular activity) and not a detector of matter/energy at the body surface. Recognizing one's hallucinations requires that logical/averaging of "sensory" conclusions by fused Is contradict those of rogue, or maverick, or malfunctioning Is. In schizophrenics, there must be an integrative fault where internal analysis and critique is unable to data average or inadequate at it. Hallucinations are accepted at face value despite other indications that the room is empty (hence no voices, monsters, creepy-crawlies, stinks or tastes).

"I" is thus a fusion of sensory inputs and the solitary motor output of brains, so that all macroscopic experiences are rendered a seamless whole. For this to materialize, "I" must consider a part of the multicellular collective to be the "I"—"non-"I" boundary .That boundary, enclosing the totality of "I," is the skin. Skin becomes, accordingly, the fused cerebral neural circuits' metaphor for the cell membrane of one-celled biota. It is not, actually, the boundary between cerebral neurons and the environment of their multicellular being, but they are obliged to consider it so , thereby rendering it a logical constant of the symbolic monitoring of and maneuvering in the macro world. Skin is metazoans' neural metaphor for the protozoan cell membrane.

If some protozoa have phototropism, that is their only long-distance sensory detection modality. All other unicellular "sensations" analogous to metazoans' involve direct contact with the cell membrane. Apposition of matter to the membrane equals metazoan "tactile" sensation and sound detection (sound causes vibratory waves in water or air, and they impact the membrane whereas it is cochlear inner ear cells that detect sound in metazoans). Molecules (detected by metazoan nasal and lingual cells to culminate in "smell" and "taste") also directly engage protozoan cell membranes. Brains, on the cuits calculate that variation has or has not occurred.

Clinically, memory is divided into immediate, intermediate and remote. The first involves retention for seconds or minutes after the event ("In 5 minutes, repeat: chalk, Devil's Island, superbowl"); the second, hours or days after ("Who won the World Series yesterday?); the last is indefinite retention (at the start of my neurologic career, Americans old enough to be unsettled by the event, were asked: "Where were you on Dec 7, 1941?"; toward the end of my career, I was asking: "What were you doing when JFK was shot?"). Symbolically, immediate memory could be the four neuron circuit below, synaptically continuing into an upstream monitor circuit:

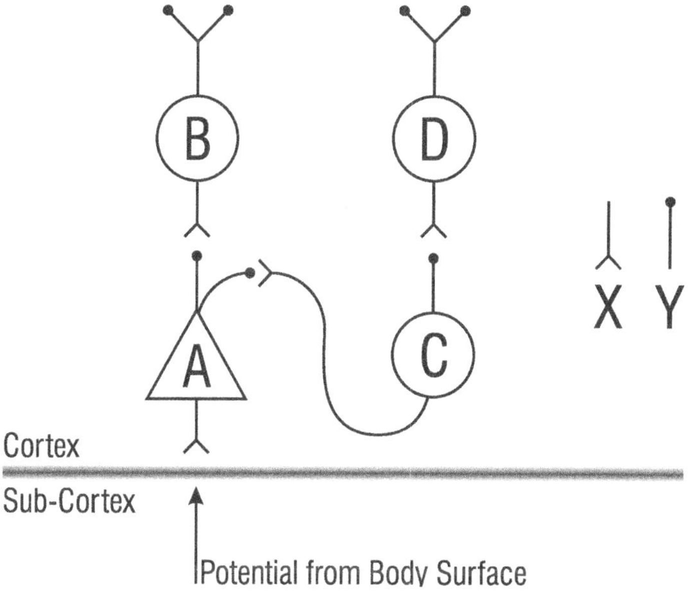

Figure 1: Immediate Memory

Here, "A" is a cortical receptor neuron varying electrically with peripheral stimulation. The variation is propagated vertically to neuron "B," which varies in turn, and horizontally to "C" causing "C" to vary. "C" synapses vertically with "D," causing bioelectric variation. Since "C" is interposed with "D," "D" varies fractionally later than "B." For the superior, monitoring circuit, the electrical states of "B" and "D" are either the same or opposites. Since "B" varies before "D," "B" equals "is" and "D," "was." Circuits superior to the monitor circuit must eventually deduce that when

IS = WAS, the environment is static, and

IS = / = WAS, the environment varies.

Since IS is now and WAS, then, variations symbolizing now occur before those symbolizing then. In the interest of symbolically processing bioelectricity, it cannot be otherwise. Present has to change before past so that monitor circuits may detect variations in time. The actual time elapsed depends on how many neurons are actually interposed between "A"—"B," "A"—"C," and "C"—"D." Whatever the case, it has to be in the millisecond range or faster. In clinical nerve conduction velocity determinations, peripheral nerve conduction velocities (e.g. median, ulnar, peroneal nerves) and central nervous system conduction velocities (brain/spinal cord, studied with evoked potentials) are of the order of 40 to 100 meters per second. In six footers, the time from stimulation of tactile sensors in the sole of the foot to variation of somatosensory neurons in the cortical foot area, is just under 0.02 (two hundredths) second. We become aware our sole was stimulated less than 0.02 seconds after. When we voluntarily curl our toes, the round trip:cerebral-command-to-muscles—arrival-of-signal-from-stimulated-muscles-to sensorimotor strip is roughly 12 feet so the latency: cerebral-command-to-muscles—muscle-response-signal-arriving-in-sensorimotor-cortex doubles to just under 0.04 sec.

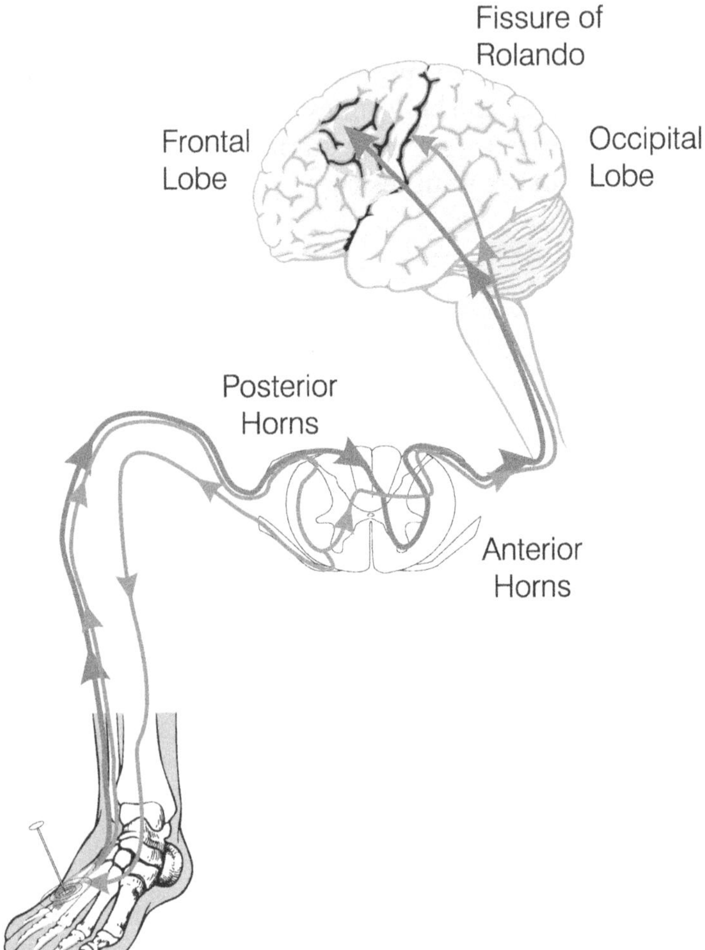

Figure 2: The Polysynaptic Reflex

In the polysynaptic reflex arc (Figure 2) skin stimulation (e.g. dorsum of foot) causes relay of bioelectric potentials to the posterior ("sensory") horn of the segmental spinal cord level which mediates electrical traffic from foot to brain and brain to foot. On entering the cord, the signal bifurcates. One route proceeds superiorly in a tract of the posterolateral cord to the brain stem, decussating to the other side and thence to a thalamic nucleus, continuing on to activate receptor neurons in the foot area of the somatosensory homunculus at the inferior, mesial portion of the postrolandic strip. The other route is transversely across the cord to the anterior (motor) horn, then in a mixed motor/sensory nerve to muscles underlying the stimulated skin area. Reflexly varying flexor/extensor muscle couples in turn relay signals signifying variation to the controlateral hemispheric sensorimotor cortex.

The only thing cerebral neural circuits can gather from the foregoing is that a first (what we know to be somatosensory receptor neuron) variation precedes, in time, a subsequent variation (which outside observers know to be sensorimotor). Cerebral neural circuits cannot know that said variations are separated in cerebral space as well as time. Nor can they know that the material items that vary are cerebral receptor neurons. Knowledge is limited to the number of variations (two) and their succession in time. Fused (integrated) neural inputs and outputs ("Is") are, however, able to register variations in all receptor cortices (a species' total "sensory" menu plus its motor strip input) and whether these are, or not, simultaneous.

In the course of self-learned muscle control, we learn to appose some parts of our body surface to others. Because of the polysynaptic reflex arc, muscles beneath stimulated skin contract reflexly whether stimulation was by non-body items as well as by other body parts. The fact that muscles varying reflexly to non-body stimuli also vary reflexly when two skin areas are brought in contact through cerebral commands to muscles, reflects the existence of an arbitrary, physical bioelectric closed loop (brain to periphery to brain) producing sequential cerebral receptor neuron variations. Symbolic breakdown and analysis of the cerebral events involving this closed loop enables neural circuits to discover the body surface, its shape and dimensions in time. The physical elements of the loop are "sensory" detectors in skin, underlying flexor/extensor muscle couples, the cortical somatosensory and motor homunculi, and pathways linking bioelectric flow in all these elements. No such loops exist for the other "sensory" modalities. The foveae (retinal regions containing light-detecting cells) cannot be juxtaposed, nor flavor and odor detectors to each other, nor the sound-detecting cells in the inner ears. None of these sensory modes includes a motor component permitting a closed loop between sensors and muscles. Therefore, the macroscopic long-range sensory modes cannot produce intracerebral neural variations with a peripheral ("sensory") and cerebral ("motor") input to "I," which logic circuits can parse so as to directly discover (define) any long-range macroscopic sensory mode. Long-range sensations cannot accordingly serve as points of departure for elaborating awareness. Their significance can be found only by reference to the previously discovered sensation, "tact." This is why research confined to the visual system (a popular stratagem among neurobiologists) cannot explain any aspect of consciousness, be it how it is elaborated or be it visual "sensation." Tactile sensation, muscle control, surface anatomy, the discovery of time and then of space are the obligatory building blocks of consciousness. IS-WAS neural circuits, and downstream circuits monitoring them must be the first in a series of progressively more complex, symbolic neural circuits constituting an ascending logic cascade. The ultimate circuits are those constituting symbolic concepts which are conclusions from logical processing of bioelectric variations. Synapses function to form circuits, equal signs (identity) between certain conclusions separated in cerebral space, and associations between other spatially separated concepts that are linked but not by identity.

Researchers focusing on the visual system describe occipital (visual cortex) cell patterns of "complex," "hyper complex" and "hyper-hyper complex" columns. Within and surrounding these are bioelectric "surround-on" and "surround-off" inhibitions. These researchers believe that understanding vision is a matter of multiplying such observations until some critical number is attained, as if observations alone are pieces of a puzzle whose global design becomes discernible when enough pieces (but not all) have been joined. I propose that "complex," "hyper-complex" and "hyper-hyper-complex" cell columns are sequential, increasingly specific symbolic cell circuits performing logical/data-averaging symbolic analysis on bioelectric variations in the striate (primary visual) cortex. Surround-on and off inhibitions are symbolic binary 1's and 0's .Understanding vision and other sensations is not a matter of making additional observations , but of decoding the symbolic significance of those available since neurons were discovered in the 1890's. This necessarily requires association pathways (fasciculi) between the somesthetic and motor homunculi and/or all cortical areas which symbolically define "tactile" sensation and control skeletal muscles. All long-range macro sensations—vision included—are rendered symbolically meaningful through logical/data averaging neural processing of bioelectric variations in the long-range cortical sensory receptor areas relative to simultaneously occurring variations in the homuncular strips.

Fusion or integration of all sensory inputs including intracortical commands to the motor strip produces several "Is" which fuse in turn, culminating in one, coherent whole experienced as "I" relative to the non-body world. "I" is a logical, symbolic variable in the ascending logic cascade culminating in consciousness. It is not the "ego" of Psychiatry, which is awareness of individuality relative to others of the species. "I" is necessary because when bioelectric potentials from skin sensors of macroscopic phenomena activate discrete somesthetic strip neurons; when, later, commands to specific skeletal muscles (believed by "I" to be limbs or segments of limbs) depart from localized neurons of the motor homunculus, symbolic processing ending with discovery of the body surface followed by learning to move parts of it, requires cerebral logic circuits to postulate that some cerebral variations are caused by me ("I"), others by non-I. Therefore, there is a non-I universe. The logical steps are as follows:

Neonatal reflexes such as the Babinski, the triple retreat, or the stereotypical outflinging of the upper extremity when palm or dorsum of hand are stimulated, reproduce activations of the distal to cephalic flexor/extensor muscle couples of limbs or segments of limbs. In triple retreat, foot muscle couples vary first, followed by muscles flexing ankle on leg, then leg on thigh, then thigh on hip. In the upper extremities, varying hand muscles are followed by forearm muscles mobilizing hand on wrist, then arm muscles mobilizing forearm on arm and finally shoulder muscles mobilizing arm relative to shoulder. The face has the root, snout and suck reflexes where stimulating any region near the mouth produces puckering of lips followed by sucking. The rationale for the facial reflexes is to enable newborns to feed. That for limb reflexes, is to withdraw limbs from potentially harmful contacts. But there is also a critically important, pedagogic rationale: the limb reflexes always cause involuntary, invariable variations of muscle couples beginning with those furthest and finishing with those nearest to the head. This produces consecutive temporal variations of areas of the sensorimotor homunculus corresponding to tail-to-head surface anatomy. Now, the somatosensory and motor homunculi are virtually superimposed in the anterior to posterior plane, those of the right hemisphere monitoring and controlling left body and those of left hemisphere, right body. In the brain, nerve tracts between the hemispheres are called commissures, tracts linking parts of a same hemisphere, fasciculi (details found in basic neurophysiologic books). By definition, pathways consist of synaptically linked neurons encased in white-matter insulation (glial cells in the brain, Schwann cells in peripheral nerves). Brains have no other recourse for forming material links symbolizing identity, or more broadly, association. Symbolically, then, some fasciculi and commissures have got to be equal signs affirming identity between two or more logical/mathematical variables, or association tracts stating some commonality between two or more concepts, e.g. dog, bark, sheep herder or sled-puller. Neurons of all sensory receptor areas might vary simultaneously to detection of aspects of a same non-body item. There must therefore exist some neural circuit mechanism, including fasciculi or physical pathways affirming commonality, which critiques and data-averages the separate sensory inputs culminating in a logical synthesis into a coherent whole. Each cerebral hemisphere monitors and exercises muscular control of the controlateral body. It is a fusion of all its sensory inputs and muscle output, each being one "I." Therefore, the fused Is of the two hemispheres must, in turn, fuse. Each species has finite sensory detector modalities and one motor output per hemisphere, so its integrated Is are numerically equal to the sum of the sensory and motor Is of each hemisphere plus the two fused Is of both. The presence of these multiple Is provides multiple physical elements for the symbolic discovery of "I": it suffices that synapses (symbolizing equality) form between some or all of them. That is, identity is established when there are at least two physical constants, and physical links symbolizing sameness form between them. And in order for the blank-slate brain to fulfill its function of elaborating consciousness by analyzing bioelectric variations within itself, there must be at least two Is, with formation of synaptic tracts symbolizing equality between them.

The purpose of brains is monitoring the macroscopic environment of metazoan organisms, and responding to it. In mobile creatures, this entails displacements which optimize survival. In immobile ones, filaments or tentacles must secure food and bring it to the mouth. "I" is required to recognize only three environmental categories: threats, vital needs, and indifferent factors. Only three types of motor response are necessary: counter threats (fight, flight, immobility, camouflage...); assimilate vital needs (secure nourishment/energy) and take no action vis a vis indifferent factors. Deciding whether a course of action is appropriate is a job for integrated Is. Neural cell circuits must therefore perform logical analyses of received, total sensory inputs each of which is a symbolic conclusion arrived at by the ascending neural logic cascade processing only that sensory modality. Each "I" incorporates cell-circuits performing logical and statistical probability assessments, data averaging and syntheses culminating in conclusions about the environment (threats, vital needs, neutral). The conclusions reached trigger bioelectric variations in circuits involved with appropriate responses to the computed environmental situation(s). It follows that "Is" have three parts: an input for all sensory modalities, a central processor containing probability and data averaging circuits, and an output for commanding variations of specific parts of the motor strip (activating specific muscles), in function of conclusions reached in the central processor. Schematically, two broad types of "I' are possible. Which type a brain has depends on the animal species, therefore on the complexity of its nervous system. The basic model consists of a largely unmodifiable sensory input section which transits I's central (logic) section virtually uncritiqued, and is channeled to the appropriate circuits of the output section (response to threat or vital need, or no response needed). Motor responses are stereotyped and invariable. The sum of sensory modality inputs (each itself a conclusion of processed bioelectric variations) goes virtually unchallenged in this sort of "I." The second, more complex "I" analyzes and critiques sensory inputs, accepting some, rejecting others. Therefore, it performs as an editor or quality comptroller of inputs. Rejected output is rerouted upstream for additional sensory processing. The result of this additional sensory processing reenters the input section and "I" a second time. If accepted, appropriate motor responses follow. This second, more sophisticated "I" therefore has either one or two outputs: a motor response in cases of inputs accepted without reservations, and the rejected inputs referred upstream for further processing. Semantically, variations returned upstream are outputs, although they "connect" with upstream logic circuits rather than with the motor-output section of "I." In cases of rejection, then, there is a first and a revised (or not) input, and two outputs: the rejected input and the final motor output. The functional import of rejected inputs is: "Check these results, send back the best conclusions."

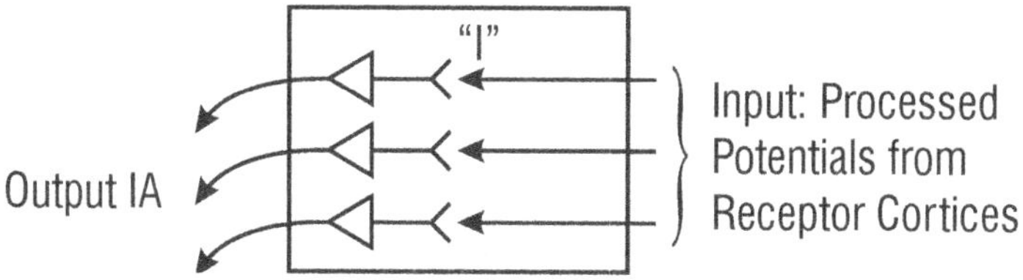

Figure 3: "I," One Input, One Output

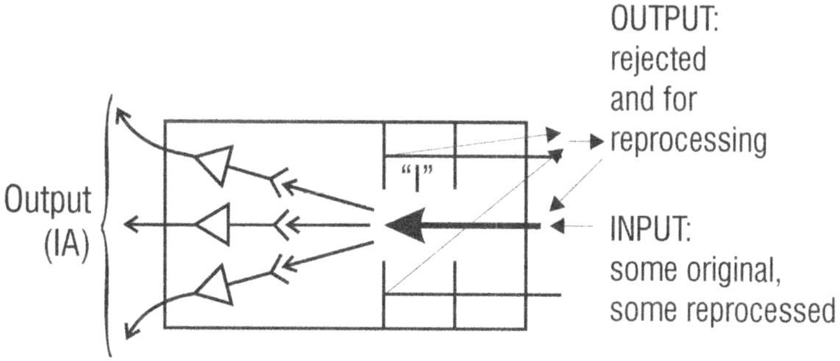

Figure 4: One Input, Two Outputs

As previously stated, two or more Is must exist in cerebral space to permit formation of synaptic links symbolizing identity. Only thus can "I" discover itself. "I" is an indispensable constant for symbolic-logical inductions concerning intracerebral bioelectric variations generated either when skeletal muscles vary reflexly due to the polysynaptic reflex arc, or to cerebral command. "I" is used as follows:

"I cause variation X.

If X occurs without my command, then there must be an agent, NON-I."

Skeletal muscles underlie precise skin areas. Spatial distances of agonist/antagonist couples from the head, and from contiguous couples closer to the head, are fixed and invariable. Absolute distances lengthen between birth and completion of body growth, but relative distances from the head and from contiguous couples remain fixed. Therefore, temporal latencies of contiguous pairs to the head remain fixed and invariable, as are the round-trip latencies: brain—muscle—brain. In the polysynaptic reflex, skin stimulation is signaled to the somesthetic homunculus behind the fissure of Rolando, and also triggers reflex contraction of underlying muscles which relay the variation to the sensorimotor homunculus. In the controlateral cerebral hemisphere, then, a first variation in the somesthetic homunculus is followed in time by a variation in the sensorimotor homunculus. But when "I" voluntarily activates skeletal muscles, there is a time zero (the departure of bioelectric potentials from the motor strip) which is analogous to the "stimulus artifact" in oscilloscopes in clinical nerve conduction studies. This "time zero" is "I's" awareness of initiating the order. It is followed in time by variations in the sensorimotor homunculus caused by signals from the varying muscle couple. "I" is not aware of the round-trip nature of these successive cerebral variations. But brains can simultaneously stimulate two or more muscle couples (we can simultaneously wiggle toes, snap fingers and whistle). Hence, "I," the integration of sensory inputs and motor output, can establish that commands to "skin" (it doesn't know the commands are to muscles below the skin) depart simultaneously (there are simultaneous "times zero") while the responses from "skin" arrive simultaneously or not. In addition, if commands to "skin" have mobilized body parts bringing some into contact, the cerebral variations caused by signals from activated muscles are followed in time by variations in the somatosensory homunculus caused by signals from cutaneous sensors in the juxtaposed areas of skin. If signals from skin stimulated by non-body agents are numbered (1), and from reflex or cerebrally activated muscles (2), and "times zero" of cerebral commands to muscles, (0): then in cases of the polysynaptic reflex, the sequence of intracerebral variations is (1)—(2)'—(2)''—(2)'''—etc when muscles vary consecutively in a tail-to-head direction. If two areas of skin involuntarily come in contact, the intracerebral sequence continues with variations (1)'—(1)''—(1)'''etc. If "I" has ordered muscle variations that have not produced contact between body parts, the cerebral variation sequence is: (0)—(2). When there results contact of body parts, the sequence in the cortex is: (0)—(2)—(1)(1)'.

Upon delivery from uteri or eggs, brains become obligated recipients of bioelectric signals from all sensors of macroscopic matter/energy. They must establish that some intracerebral variations are signals from a periphery, plot its morphology and dimensions, and learn to activate skeletal muscle (which brains believe are portions of the body surface) in some logical, immutable order.

Metazoans pass infancy and childhood learning basic muscle control. Some spend lifetimes fine-tuning and specializing at this: musicians, sculptors and painters, the numerous athletic disciplines etc. At birth, the human brain contains all the gray ("thinking") cells it will have. Yet it virtually triples in volume by age 2 or 3. This increase is due to formation of additional white matter (glia, or non-thinking cells). Some of these (astrocytes) were recently shown to be indispensable in forming synapses between neurons (gray cells)[3].

"...Few synapses form in the absence of glial cells and the few synapses that do form are functionally immature. Astrocytes increase the number of mature, functional synapses on central nervous system (CNS) neurons by sevenfold and are required for synaptic maintenance in vitro...most synapses are generated concurrently with the development of glia in vivo. These data demonstrate a previously unknown function for glia in inducing and stabilizing CNS synapses."

Gray cells are essentially non-renewable. Their loss is irreversible. Glia, including astrocytes, are replaceable. In non-tumor situations, however, the total amount of white matter stays constant after a critical volume is reached. This happens around 2 or 3 years of age in humans, as judged by comparison of infant and adult brains on MRI, autopsy studies, and major cognitive attainments. Past this age, sensations do not develop for the first time. Therefore, in average, healthy humans the major neural circuits and networks involved in elaborating sentience must have formed by 2-3 years of age. Non-formation by this deadline (which corresponds to completion of cerebral myelination) is incompatible with acquisition of sensory modalities. This must explain why

3. "*Control of Synapse Number* by Glia"' E.M. Ullian, S.K. Sapperstein et al, Science, Vol. 291 No. 5504, 26 Jan. 2001, pp 657-659:

repair of damaged/infected/malfunctioning sense organs, or of muscle imbalance (maintaining binocular fixation on the same object through the six extra ocular muscles of each eye) allows sensations to develop whereas repair after the deadline cannot produce a sensory modality at all, or produces a defective one. Thus, strabismus (where incoordination of eye muscles prevents binocular fixation on the same target) may be corrected at any age by eye muscle surgery. But surgery performed after 3-5 years of age will not lead to acquiring depth perception. Surgery or patching the good eye before then (forcing the bad eye to focus on targets) yields stereopsis. If congenital cataracts go untreated, there is congenital blindness. The concept of light never forms. But cataract surgery done before the deadline age allows elaboration of visual "sensation" In like vein, early, untreated inner ear problems (e.g. infections) prevent acquisition of hearing, of the concept of sound and of spoken language. But cochlear implants before the deadline age allow elaboration of greater or lesser degrees of auditory "sensation." The inference from all this is that cell circuits fundamental for elaborating sensation must have formed by the time of completion of cerebral myelination (2-3 years of age) and cannot form afterward. At the microscopic level, synapses fundamental in building awareness have to form during this critical period of white matter build-up, culminating in specific circuits; also, between some of these circuits, constituting symbolic equal signs or association tracts, in the form of fasciculi and commissures. Recall that the former link regions within one cerebral hemisphere, the latter, regions in each hemisphere. A pathologic instance of intrahemispheric linkage is "kindling:" the formation of a secondary epileptic focus in the hemisphere controlateral to that containing the original focus of electrical abnormality. Given time, some secondary foci become more active than the original, complicating pharmacologic control of the epilepsy. We are led to conclude that in normal circumstances, fasciculi symbolizing sameness or identity must form between homologous regions of the somesthetic and sensorimotor homunculi, as well as their supplementary areas (secondary and tertiary). This is the physical scaffold permitting brains to discover the existence of a body surface, and to learn to mobilize parts of that surface.

Now, think about latencies (times elapsed from onset of an electrical potential at a point in space, to its arrival at another point). In the polysynaptic reflex, there is a first latency corresponding to signals from skin sensors triggered by contact (time one) and arrival in the somatosensory homunculus. Brains register only the arrival, which they learn to recognize as: a portion of skin was "touched." Soon after, there arrives in the sensorimotor homunculus, the potential from reflex varying muscles under the area of skin that was "touched." Eventually, brains learn to activate specific muscles. A muscle varying to cerebral command gives brains both the time zero of a latency and its temporal end, because "I" registers the instant of command (time zero) and the later arrival, in the cortex, of the potential emitted when the muscle couple varied (temporal duration of the latency). Brains don't know that a round trip is involved. But brain—muscle—brain latencies are invariable for specific muscle couples, and brains have all the time to register same latencies repeatedly, and invariable differences in latency of specific muscle couples (believed to be skin), also repeatedly. When all latencies, and the differences between them, have been registered, round-trip brain—skin—brain latencies may be registered, again sans awareness by "I" that a round trip is involved. For cerebral commands to muscles can in some cases bring areas of skin in apposition. When this occurs, there is an intracerebral time zero (the command to muscles) and an intracerebral end of the latency: the arrival, in two homuncular areas, of signals from juxtaposed regions of skin. The two signals arrive in the same homunculus when the parts in contact are on the same side of the body (right thumb on right thigh) or in each homunculus when the "touching" parts are controlateral (right thumb-left thigh). There is, then, a brain—muscle—skin—brain loop where bioelectric variations consecutive in time all occur intracerebrally. That is why brains can initiate the analyses culminating in awareness. No such loops exist for the macroscopic long-range senses, rendering them logically unsuitable as points of departure of analyses of intracerebral variations culminating in sentience. Elaborating any long-range macroscopic sensation is entirely contingent on first elaborating "tact" and a "body image."

As argued above, when brains mobilize muscles producing apposition of body parts, they are unaware that time zero of the latency (the command from the motor strip) activates muscles (brains believe they send signals to limb segments, or to elephants' trunks, or to eyes, or to cats' tails, not to muscles in these structures). They learn that signals from apposed body parts are from skin, but the time-zero variations and the variations produced in the somesthetic homunculus (that brains are not aware of) are, each, intracortical. Brains are not aware of the round-trip nature of the brain—muscle—two skin areas loop. But when brains order several muscle couples to vary simultaneously, (say foot, thumb and lip muscles) they know they register that the orders (times zero of the latencies) are simultaneous, and that signals from activated foot, thumb, and lip areas appear simultaneously or not. When signals from different areas appear staggered in time (or simultaneously) the temporal differences for two or more same areas are constant, invariable and reproducible. Somewhere in cerebral space, a registry of muscle (areas of the corporal envelope, to "I") latencies must form. They do not vary over time—at least, not relative to each other. Healthy newborn brains have no choice but to receive latencies (more correctly, to initiate those latencies rendered possible by the closed-loop brain—somatosensory—muscle—brain wiring). It is reasonable to postulate that registries of same, recurrent variations (significance to be worked out) are established for somesthesia as well as for muscles. They have invariable upper and lower limits (distance in time, from heads, of toe and scalp muscles). Neural cell circuits symbolically performing mathematical interpolations and later extrapolations must posit horizontal and vertical axes and construct a temporal plot of the body surface from these latencies. The shortest and longest latencies, and all latencies in-between, represent distances in time (converted, in a second logical phase, into space) of muscles ("body-surface parts") from "I" (the head). (see Figure 7 on page 100.)

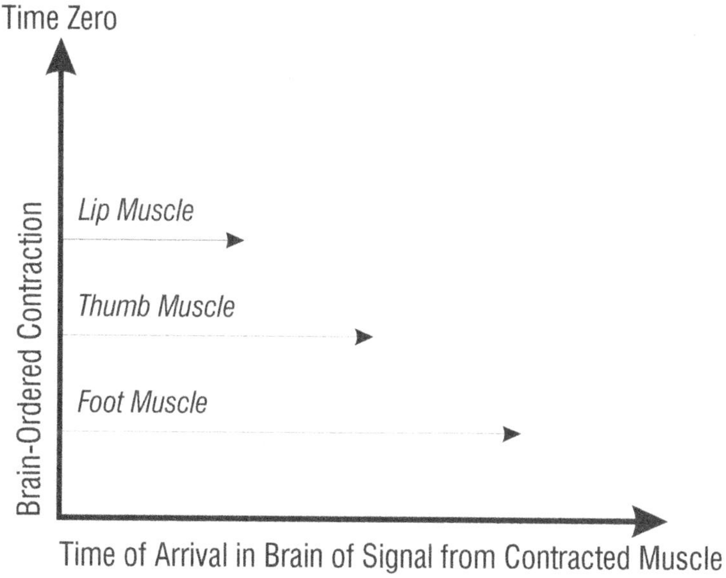

Chronologic Latencies: Different arrival times in brain, when muscles were ordered to contract simultaneously.

Figure 5: Chronologic Latencies

Let us now develop, in detail, the hypothesis that some synaptic links (fascicular or commissural) must symbolize sameness-equality-identity. For cerebral neurons to ensure survival of multicellular beings in the macroscopic world, they must discover the being first, then the non-being world, by processing intracerebral bioelectric variations. They must discover, identify and interact with macroscopic matter/energy. They discover time in a first logical operation, and space next. For cerebral neural nets, time/space is the matrix of the universe, matter so many reliefs on that matrix. Logically and mathematically the formulae needed to pinpoint reliefs and their location on the matrix are interpolation and extrapolation formulae—the very ones taught in school. They are symbolic neural circuits in cerebral space. Within circuits, bioelectric variations are symbolically meaningful. Data and devices collecting data for neural circuit processing is relatively undifferentiated, non-specific and general. Any device triggered by matter/energy suffices. Relatively few triggering modalities are needed. Signals may be relayed however the system allows, and funneled through a series of neural circuits symbolically processing electrical variations in the cortex, concluding (a) that data is being received and (b) it signifies variations in detectors of macro matter/energy. It is a fact that "sense organs" constantly vary in response to stimuli by non-body phenomena and also by apposed body surface parts. Portions of skin contact each other, or there is non-body-skin contact, or no contact. Non-contact is fundamentally necessary for organs registering light, sound, or molecules reflected or emitted from surfaces. Detection and localization always involve surfaces. The three-dimensional relief (shape) of encountered matter is derived by multiplying individual contacts so as to establish the curvature of plotted points. Mathematically, plotting the spatial boundaries of surfaces starts with determination of their polar coordinates.

The next step is fitting the coordinates to a set of axes seving as absolute reference-points. The axes available to brains as reference-points for non-body polar coordination of matter, are those of the body surface, previously plotted by neural circuits. They are derived by logical/mathematical interpolation. The non-body world is registered and plotted relative to the axes of the body. Accordingly, the point of departure in building consciousness is the neuronal deduction (a necessary hypothesis) that multicellular bodies are details (reliefs) projected on a time/space matrix (continuum).The next, necessary step in constructing awareness from bioelectric variations inside the head, is plotting the axes and polar coordinates of the corporal envelope. That is interpolation. It is followed by extrapolating items of the non-body world from these axes. Logically and mathematically, then, the broad outline of chronologic cognitive development is

Interpolation: discovering (plotting) the body surface

a. computing the functional relation of data sets (more on set theory later).
b. computing the functional significance of data.
c. computing the axes of the body (polar coordination).
d. computing the surface of the body (curve fitting).

Extrapolation: discovering (computing) the environment by reference to the polar coordinates (axes) of the body.

Returning, now to the hypothesis that some synaptic links symbolize identity: if this is true, there have to be two or more “Is,” because the “brain” can search only itself to find "I." To make the discovery, synapses must form between all Is.

Let "I" be defined as at least two or more neocortical autoregulatory circuits consisting of the fusion of all sensory inputs and motor outputs, in separate loci of cerebral space, fused in turn by the formation of fascicular or commissural synaptic tracts symbolizing identity. "I" is relatively autonomous because its input is mostly neocortical. In some circumstances, however, both its input and output can be usurped by the autonomic (vegetative) nervous system. Examples are being paralyzed with fright, trembling uncontrollably with fear, losing sphincter control with fear etc. "I" is only semiautonomous because it functions only during wakefulness. During sleep, its sensory inputs are seriously curtailed and it does not maneuver the multicellular collective in response to all monitored circumstances. What evidence can be mustered for the existence of "I"?

Fact: Obviously, "I" is itself a circuit system analogous in many ways to other circuits discussed in this book—but subject matter for a book of its own. The objective of *this* book is discovery of the nature and construction of cognition and mind, for which the synaptic cross-indexing of "I" is critical. We are not trying to reason out the circuitry of "I." what evidence can we muster for "I"?

Fact: During sleep the full exercise of "I" is curtailed. Monitoring and interacting with the macro world are curtailed or inoperative. "I" operates at low intensity or not at all. Short of death, the ultimate non-activity of the auto regulator occurs in coma. But the reverse can occur. Somewhere between the hypothalamus and brainstem is a cluster of neurons called the "sleep center." Destroying this center or its outflow tract restricts sleep or abolishes it altogether. This is usually seen in some war injuries. Some of the injured never sleep. The significance of this documented phenomenon is that it is *pathological.* Perpetually full-intensity "I" operation happens only accidentally or through interference with the sleep center or its outflow tract. Normally and despite all attempts to stay awake, "I" is always "KO'd" by the sleep center. The center is *not* neocortical but *autonomic*—and it is the autonomic nervous system which *arouses* "I," by means of a formation called the "reticular activating system."

Fact: "I's" of awake individuals may be pushed aside, and their neocortices taken control of (continuing to function despite "I"), by another part of the neocortex which is *not* an "I" circuit, in the condition termed "psychomotor epilepsy." There are several forms of epilepsy, each characterized by abnormal electrical activity, more or less sustained, of a part or more than one part of the brain. Behavioral manifestations depend on the area or areas which are abnormally active. Thus, if a focus of abnormal electric discharges is confined to part or all of a motor strip, the sufferer experiences convulsions of muscles of the controlateral body which are normally interoactivated by "I"—i.e., normally only "I' gives intracerebral orders (stimulates) to neurons of the motor strip. The epileptic non-"I" focus may be in the motor strip or not. If it is not, it stimulates neurons in the strip synaptically. The victim stays awake and cognizant of his jerking limbs but the IA tract linking "I" with the stimulated motor strip neurons has been short-circuited. Pathological foci of bioelectricity have seized control of the motor strip from "I" and the victim is powerless to control the convulsions. In the "sensory" epilepsies, neurons of the neuronal sensory receptor areas or their downstream circuits (IS-WAS; association circuits) are stimulated by non-"I" foci (obviously! We command our muscles, but not our sensations!) in the receptor cortices or synaptically from outside said cortices. Victims experience the *illusion* that the peripheral organs activating the stimulated cortical neurons *were* activated, which is not the case—the peripheral organs are *not* stimulating the abnormally active neurons. If the receptor cortex is the somesthetic cortex or a circuit downstream from same, then the individual might experience a pins-and-needles sensation of the skin area normally stimulating the abnormally discharging cortical neurons. If the malfunctioning cortex is occipital cortex number 17 (the striate cortex) people "see" flashes, dots, stars, or lights. Should only the auditory cortex be active, people will "hear" unusual sounds or noises and similarly for the olfactory and gustatory receptor cortices. So long as consciousness is preserved, victims know they are hallucinating because their "I" editors, receiving simultaneous inputs from *all* indices, are aware that no other "sensory" system corroborates the "report" by the malfunctioning system. Should pathologic discharges spread to all areas of the brain, then the arousal center (the reticular activating system) will be turned off. The epileptic will lapse into coma, but since his motor strips are being activated along with other parts of the brain ("I" and the arousal center being, however, deactivated) he will have tonic-clonic convulsions. There are other varieties of epilepsy, but that which is relevant to our discussion is (in the old terminology) psychomotor epilepsy. The signature of a psychomotor seizure (partial complex seizure in current terminology) is automatic, stereotypical behavior. For a given individual, the behavior is usually the same for every seizure. To onlookers the behavior seems purposeful but not goal-directed. It may consist of lip-smacking, chewing, humming, fiddling with clothes, attacks of unprovoked rage, etc. Consciousness is retained unless the reticular activating system is knocked out. If not, people continue driving, climbing stairs, walking, and so on. Usually they don't answer when addressed, but this varies in degree. What strikes spectators is the total irrelevance of the behavior in the actual circumstances the stricken individual is in.

In psychomotor seizures the functional role of "I" is partially usurped by one or more foci of pathological electrical activity. Monitoring and interacting with the world are ongoing, but neither is entirely consistent with the circumstances of the time. The importance of the foregoing is that if we recognize, admit, *know* that there are cases of *abnormal* activation of the motor strip and/or other brain areas by pathologic foci (some of them outside the afflicted area(s)), then there must be *normal* cerebral activators of these areas and an intracerebral beneficiary of processed potentials received in the neocortex from sense organs which were actually triggered at the periphery. This intracerebral beneficiary is also the *normal* intracerebral activator of the motor strip. The beneficiary of actual sensory data and activator of the motor strip in function of it is the neuronal auto regulator or "I." Now, it was postulated earlier that the neuronal declaration of identity is the cross-indexing synapse. There must therefore exist at least two indices having the functional significance, "I." The possibilities are: Two or more indices each *explicitly* signifying "I"; one which is explicit and others which are only functionally explicit; none which are explicit but all which are implicitly significant, and (since there are two cerebral hemispheres) some variation of these possibilities. And, the indices must be cross-indexed. Remember why this is necessary: it must be so in order to be able to deduce: "I cause x; therefore if x occurs sans me, then the cause is non-me." "I" must somehow discover itself (i.e. establish its own identity by cross-indexing) and that is possible only if there be a minimum of two cross-indexed registries. "I" is a logical or mathematical variable in a chain of logic. Its existence is indispensable to neuronal data processing, but it is *not* synonymous with awareness of macroscopic individual self.

Decades ago, I came across this "definition" in a book of jokes: "Silence is what you don't hear when you listen." Rendered in specialist's jargon but no less naïve, this becomes: "Silence is non-activation of the auditory system" (cochlear cells, cerebral auditory receptor neurons and downstream circuits). The naiveté is due to not specifying: "Provided there is the concept of sound." For "silence" means total absence of sound. Total absence is a negative concept signifying: non-sound. Those with *acquired* deafness lead "lives of silence." The universe contains a phenomenon called "sound." Brains may at best substitute a *symbol* for the phenomenon—they cannot contain actual sound. "Silence" is the neuronal deduction that the world is in a state of *non-sound* made inside brains which are monitoring the environment, which already possess the concept of sound and which benefit from a functioning auditory system. In the logical statement, "If x then non-x," "x" must exist, or be demonstrable, in order to justify the hypothesis of "non-x." The reverse is not logically defensible—one cannot affirm that "x" exists because "non-x" does (the fallacy of the word "atheist"). In other words, "silence" is the computation by a system capable of registering and *indexing* auditory potentials (whose meaning was previously deduced by that system) that registration and indexing are not occurring, although the system is actively monitoring (primed for activation). It is a referential or relative concept: non-sound. All non-x variables are logically sustainable only by reference to neuronal "X" concepts, the relation being materially made by a synapse—and this applies to "I"—"non-I" as it does to all such cases. Without a frame of reference (literally, a symbolic neuronal "I" registry) how does "I" discover "I"?

Note that there is no mysticism, nor metaphysics in this concept of "I." We are searching for explicit synaptic liaisons between explicit, functioning neuronal circuits. And, because I have the analytical bit in my teeth, I allow myself some analytical license and modify my first definition of "I," to wit:

Second definition: "I" is that component of the neuronal auto regulator which I call the "editor." it is more-or-less developed (or rudimentary) in both humans and non-humans. Inadequate human "I's" yield psychiatric pathologies, while the sophistication of animals' "I's" determines how well their brains will deal with the macro world. As to how the identity (i.e. synaptic cross-indexing) of "I's" actually appears in brains, and how it evolves, I propose the following. First, the principles of neuronal data processing as I presently see them:

Principle #1: All signals and all data of identical meaning are received and grouped in distinct brain areas.

Principle #2: Neurons of receptor cortices are organized in circuits. Received signals are rendered symbolic in some binary, decimal or other "language."

Principle #3: Relations between data sets are established through routing to progressive downstream circuits consisting of immediate memory (IS-WAS), "monitor" and "discriminator" circuits, of the symbols generated in the primary cortical receptor cortices. The products of the monitor/discriminator circuits are functionally related symbols (i.e. different symbols of different sensory modalities concerning the same environmental item) of different data sets, grouped in indices, whose meaning *may* be established by passage through a series of logic gates. The *key* to processing through the logic gates is possession of the variable, "I." The sine qua non for deducing the existence of the non-body world is the deduction: "I cause x. If x occurs without me, then non-me causes x."

Principle #4: All neuronal activity of identical functional significance is grouped in distinct brain areas. This applies to neurons activated from within the brain as well as those activated by signals from the body.

Principle #5: Therefore, when "I" activates the motor strip it must, via collateral axons, relay potentials simultaneously to a neuronal interoactivation immediate-memory (or: IA IS-WAS) area. Potentials received therein *must* be processed through the monitor/discriminator circuit chain exactly like potentials received from outside the brain. The result is a neuronal "commands by 'I'," or: "I"-command, or, more simply: Interoactivation (IA) index, interoactivation understood to be by "I." (FIG 6 —IA IS-WAS INDEX)

Principle #6: *"I" was, itself, induced.* It was formed by potentials relayed from the autonomic brain. These culminated in more than one "I" indices, making possible synaptic cross-indexing and thus self-identification, setting in motion the logic cascade culminating in computation of the body surface and non-body universe.

The mechanism whereby "I" relays potentials to a neuronal Interoactivation—IS-WAS receptor area (tantamount to an "I"—immediate-recall receptor strip) has got to be the previously described axonal splitting of signals to different destinations. Forked axons route commands to the motor strip (interoactivation) *and* to a primary neuronal IA-IS-WAS receptor cortex. The rationale for this hypothesis is the fact of being the monitors of our own actions and being able to remember initiating them. That is, remembering what we ordered our muscles to do requires the presence, somewhere in cerebral space, of immediate and intermediate recall areas for self-willed muscle activity (or self-willed muscle variations, since the variables monitored by neuronal circuits are variations of electrical states of other cerebral neurons). Diagrammatically (Figure 6) the motor output tract from “I” must be bifurcated. One terminal activates neurons in the motor strip. They, in turn, have a bifurcated output: one terminus leads to the neuromuscular junction stimulating designated muscles, and the other terminal leads to an interoactivation immediate recall (IS-WAS) area. The other terminal of the bifurcated “I” motor output lead to an “’I’-IA-IS-WAS” area. Since it is at least one synapse shorter than “IA-IS-WAS,” it varies *before* IA-IS-WAS and downstream logic gates may compute that “I” induced (or ordered) IA. Schematically:

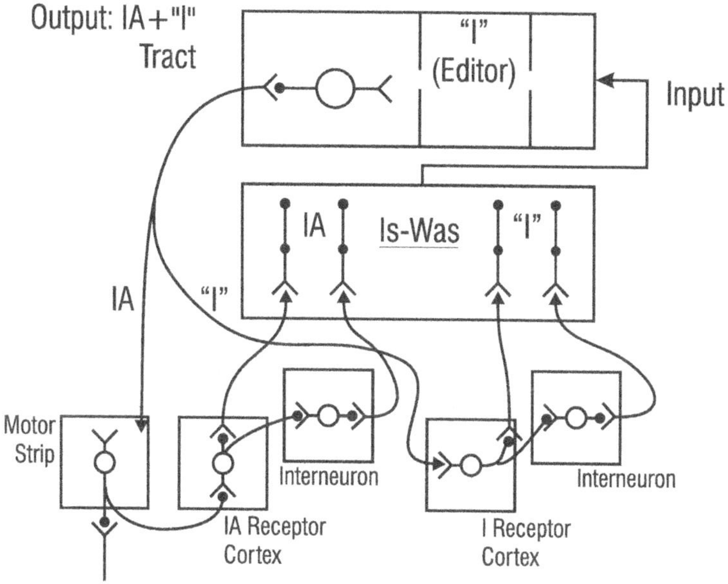

Figure 6: IA and "I" Receptor Areas

Some version of this arrangement must exist and "predict" the "wiring" for intermediate and long-range memories. Sans same there could be no language, historiography, autobiography, or literature including the genre containing the question, "What were you doing on…?" Researchers have shown that, as in primary and "supplementary" sensory areas, so too there are one primary and at least one secondary motor strips in each cerebral hemisphere. I submit that the "secondary" motor area may in fact be the interoactivation receptor cortex (functionally equivalent to "I") and the tertiary motor strip is the activated-motor-neuron memory area. The secondary motor cortex, is the immediate recall of "I's" commands to the motor strip, and the tertiary cortex is the immediate memory of activations of neurons in the motor strip, analogous to "I" to the stimulus artifact on the oscilloscope in clinical nerve conduction velocity studies. As to how "I" establishes its own identity: I have argued that its autonomy is relative, conditional and partial vis a vis the autonomic nervous system.

Principle #7: The autonomic brain induces the neocortical neuronal autoregulator ("I"). Since all potentials received in the neocortex are grouped in spatial data sets, those from the autonomic brain to "I" are addressed explicitly *to* it in a manner to be shown. Since all arrivals are indexed (at least once) "I" has merely to establish by cross-indexing that "to 'I'" means: to itself. This is how it discovers its identity.

To explain this properly, we must return to the matter of cognitive phylogenesis. It is logically reasonable to assume that if supra-autonomic "I's" exist—an incontrovertible fact or "I" could not write this nor "you" read it—then there must be an autonomic "I." Protoplasm is, after all, only matter/energy which is *functionally and mathematically* demarcated from inert matter/energy comprising most matter of the universe. We have seen that there is a microscopic or quantal or unicellular and molecular order of cognition, and a macroscopic or *aggregate* order. The "I" we are studying belongs to the latter. But functionally, phylogenetically, embryologically and in terms of comparative zoology the macro "I" cannot be dissociated from the cellular. Phylogenetically, the quantal order preceded the macro because the first living organisms were microscopic. And, a cursory inspection of contemporary animalia suggests that in many animals the quantal order remains the only "I" and that in non-humans with brains it utterly dominates neopallial "I."

At this juncture it is apropos to ask how one decides whether particular multicellular aggregates are individual organisms or colonies of discreet individuals. This is relevant because there can be so doubt that each of us has at *least* two "I" circuits. For, except for rare individuals who had an entire cerebral hemisphere resected in early life (a last recourse in unilateral, intractable epilepsy) most of us function with two hemispheres. Each hemisphere must have at least one "I," and since potentials (i.e. data) are exchanged between the hemispheres via several commisures, each "I" can monitor the other. Since the functional significance of "I" outputs is: auto regulation, each "I" "observes" something which is functionally identical to itself. It is as if whenever we are awake, we contemplate our mirror image—what we do and how. I do not propose this as the only, or even principal way "I" establishes its identity. Remember my previous hypothesis of several possible "I" index *categories*, implicit or explicit, any combination of which may lead to discovering "I" by means of synaptic cross-indexing. The facts of normal intellect and control of one's body following early resection of a cerebral hemisphere suggest that each hemisphere has at least two "I" indices. I want to forestall objections that having more than one "I" *necessarily* implies schizophrenia. It is probable that having several "I's" makes schizophrenia possible, but the condition is (by definition) pathological. Normal people are not schizophrenic despite their several I's. Some might object that only one "I" regulates both hemispheres because duplication complicates life. The argument would be made that while the hemispheres have common features, each also is specialized. The speech command center is in the left hemisphere in the majority of the population, spatial abstraction, orientation and mathematics are right-sided in most people. Accordingly, why shouldn't there be a single auto regulator for both hemispheres, located in just one? The answer is, that a single "I" cannot be cross-indexed so as to establish its identity. In a fantasy world this might be unnecessary, but in the real world products composed of specific parts cannot spring into existence by spontaneous generation. The frame of reference for "I" is (and can only be) at least one other "I." There is simply no way of establishing synaptic identity sans this other "I." I venture that each hemisphere has an "I," and they monitor each other. Each can discover itself independently of the other. Mutual surveillance might accelerate self-identification but is not the primary self-identification mechanism (as I shall show). Normally, we are not schizophrenic because our I's are fused. One supports this claim by appealing to the clinical entity of split brains. In split brains the hemispheres cannot exchange information. The condition is the paradigm of the saying: the right hand doesn't know what the left is doing (actually, neither *hemisphere* does). Yet these people are not schizophrenic if they weren't so before their commissurotomies.

To grasp why it is logically necessary that there be at least two cross-indexed Is, consider bi or polyglottism. Theorem: The material channels of computer cross-indexing and biologic synaptic cross-indexing, *may*, in appropriate cases, correspond to the mathematical equality symbol (=)—i.e., to *identity*.

In mathematics identity is expressed by the general formula, X = Y.

In logic, identity is the statement: X is materially equivalent to Y, symbolized as: X ≡ Y.

In seemingly spontaneous, unrehearsed circumstances (a fallacy—neuronal dynamic events and bioelectric latencies and conduction velocities produce all cognitive "spontaneity")—it is the exclamation: X is the same as Y.

In the actual, arbitrary world which must be discovered and described by empirical mathematics (see Appendix on page 167), *every* identity *requires* familiarity with, or experience of, one of the two variables (X or Y). Familiarity or experience of one variable *may*, with additional and *appropriately processed* data, culminate in establishment of a synaptic equality (=) link. Histologically then, some—but not all—synapses are equal signs.

To illustrate this notion, consider bilingualism and polylingualism. What happens in the neocortex when we learn a new language?

When first encountering new languages we already have auditory (and if we are literate, visual) data banks of spoken and written vocabularies of our native tongue. Our neocortex contains indices of neuronal variations grouped by a neocortical "discriminator circuit"—variations of neurons in the auditory receptor cortex triggered by signals from cochlear hair cells of the inner ear stimulated by particular frequencies (cycles per second) of sound. These frequencies were emitted by controlled vibrations of someone's vocal cords. These particular variations had been rendered meaningful by neuronal association circuits, a variant of cross-indexing. We only *assume* that native tongues come "naturally"—neuronal work was our lingual builder, and spontaneous generation is a theory conclusively disproved by Louis Pasteur. We possess another index of neuronal variations previously determined to be meaningful by association circuits: neuronal variations in the visual (occipital) receptor cortex whenever light from a line of print stimulates our retinal rods and cones. In non-mute, non-deaf people visual and spoken language indices are cross-indexed because spoken language was used to *induce* literacy.

Now, we begin being exposed to the new language. If exposure is exclusively aural, we are either told or find on our own that particular sound-frequency variations of our own auditory receptor neurons (activated from our cochlear cells stimulated by those frequencies) correspond to things we have previously encountered and indexed in the spoken-language registry of our native tongue. Say you don't speak French and the sound-frequency combination "maison" crops up while someone points at a "maison." After several recurrences your association circuits will establish that "maison" is a man-made edifice for habitation which is an item in the spoken and written indices of your native language contained in your neocortex. A new spoken-language index begins to be elaborated: Chapter heading, *Data set*: French; Sub-set: Auditory (or: Spoken). As you compute the functional significance of particular, recurrent sound frequencies causing particular cortical auditory receptor neuron variations the index grows, for example:

maison
chanter
arbre
disputer
main

Now, *mathematically* "hearing" is a data category or set: those variations of activity of cortical receptor neurons in Heschl's gyri of the temporal lobes induced by non-contact (i.e. non-tactile), non-vision, non-gustatory, or olfactory stimulation of detectors of a particular form of matter/energy: the ears. Schematically, hearing (H) is materially non-tact, non-vision, non-olfaction, and non-gustation or: $H = \sim C, \sim V, \sim O, \sim G$.

Let m be the element of the "hearing" data set "maison," c = "chanter," a = "arbre," d = "disputer" etc. The index is *actually* an arrangement of cortical neurons having specific meaning, and the symbolic arrangement is:

$$A = \begin{array}{l} m \sim C, V, \sim O, \sim G \\ c \sim C, V, \sim O, \sim G \\ a \sim C, \sim V, \sim O, \sim G \\ d \sim C, \sim V, \sim O, \sim G \end{array}$$

Read: That m variable of the A data set corresponding to non-C, non-V, non-O, non-G when the external item induces simultaneous variations of auditory, somesthetic, visual, olfactory, and gustatory cortical receptor neurons. And similarly for c, a, and d.

Since it is cumbersome to draw such "real" indices, we will continue with word-indices for convenience's sake. You begin elaborating an "H" (for hearing, or auditory) index of non-body items as symbolized in French—spoken French, which induces specific cortical auditory neuron receptor variations. But you *already* possess an "H" index of these items—in your native tongue. However, it is unlikely that you learn French words in precisely the order you learned their synonyms in your native language. If that language is English, establishing precise synaptic links (i.e. cross-indexing) between French and English elements of the "H' data sets (or indices) will entail intricate and convoluted "wiring" in three dimensions. A hint of this intricacy and complexity is given in two dimensions as follows:

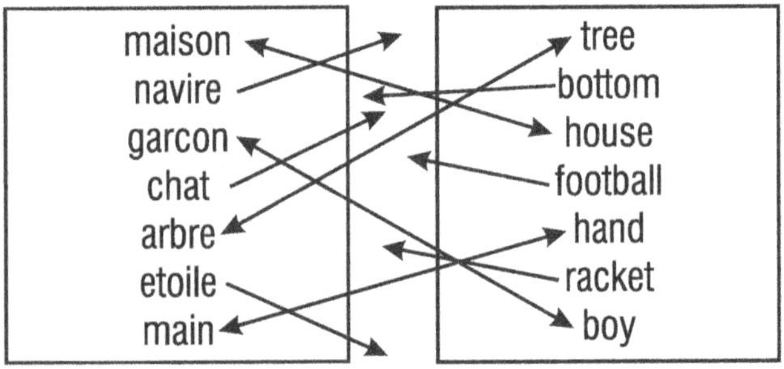

Many people are inept at mastering now languages after childhood. Herein lies part of the explanation. Consider that auditory cross-indexing intricacy is magnified if there exist, also, written-word registries in both languages and thus two cross-indexed written-word registries with each other and with each spoken-word registry. Say you also speak Hebrew.

Intricacy increases further. Merely for the written word, for example:

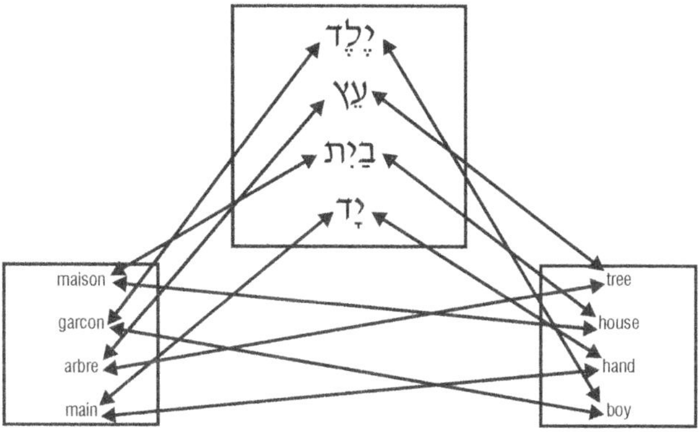

The intent of the preceding discussion is to show that at the microscopic, symbolic level identity, or equal signs, or (to be specific) the cross-indexing synapse might not form although one variable is familiar. In such cases one speculates that non-referenced variables are obliterated or stored as unknowns in the expectation of someday becoming cross-indexed. One is in the familiar situation of knowing one is hearing a non-native language, and even which language it is, yet having not a glimmer of understanding what the other man is saying. It is possible to know that one is hearing French without appreciating the meaning of the registered sounds.

Identity (or mathematical "equality" or "material equivalence" in logic) is therefore a physical, material organic *thing*: a cross-indexing synapse between two members of two data sets whose meaning is the same. Given neuronal indexing of data with "a" in one set and "b" in another, and if the meaning of either of them is established, then synaptic linkage of the two constitutes, ipso facto, equivalence or: identity. The cross-indexing synapse constitutes functional identity. But it is possible to *register* an unknown variable in a data set yet fail to form a synaptic liaison with an indexed element of another set whose meaning is established. Thus that which is familiar (whose functional significance was computed) might be of no use in interpreting a newly registered neuronal variation signifying the same thing, in cases of non-formation or of misdirection of synaptic cross-indexing. In brief, it is possible to establish identity between two or more neuronal variations concerning a same non-body item, when both or all are registered and indexed and at least one was discovered to be meaningful. But *simply* registering two or more neuronal variations concerning same items, although necessary, is insufficient to ensure that identity (in the form of a cross-indexing synapse) will be established.

It thus seems that if we are to discover the "I" circuit, we must look for two or more synaptically cross-indexed registries, each signifying "I."

Each cortical area activated by potentials from peripheral detectors of matter/energy is a data set because signals concern only one aspect of the macro environment: light in the occipital lobes, sound in the posterior temporal operculum, pressures, textures, temperature in the somatosensory strip behind the fissure of Orlando, etc. Functionally, the prerolandic motor strip is a data set of cerebral signals stimulating muscles. The justification for this assertion is the fact that animals must learn to control "voluntary" muscles. We have previously noted the learning sequence, and the relative duration of phases, for humans, deer and antelopes. Discovering that some intracortical electric variations are signals, and that signal modalities are few and discrete, requires formation of association, averaging and probability-determining circuits, possibly others too. Neocortical volume is finite, maximal size being reached in early childhood. Space limitations impose wiring constraints because of the sheer quantity of operations needed to reach valid conclusions and the numbers and types of circuits needed for step-by-step simultaneous processing of multifactorial incoming signals. Think how complicated and error-prone synaptic formation would be if cerebral neurons stimulating muscles in the left thumb adjoined neurons receiving signals from red-reflecting objects in the right superior temporal visual field, themselves adjoining neurons which receive signals concerning sound in the 1000-1100Hz range, etc. Each modality in this scenario occupies a fixed cerebral location, but the risks of synaptic snags are astronomical. Collecting all signals concerning a single aspect of the world in one cortical area minimizes the risks of synaptic snarls. In humans, six such primary collections are needed: occipital (area 17 or the striate cortex) for signals of light in the ROYGBIV (red-orange-yellow-green-blue-indigo-violet) bands, sound in the temporal lobes for roughly 500-17,000 Hz, skin mechano/temperature detectors in the postrolandic "somesthetic" strip and similarly for environmental molecules ("smell" and "taste"). The sixth neocortical data collection locus is the motor strip which is a *receptor* area because the activators of specific neuronal variations in the strip are neocortical and autonomic, i.e. cerebral neurons rather than remote "sense organs" at the body surface separated from their receptor cortices by peripheral and central nervous system neurons which propagate their potentials when triggered by their specific stimulus. The "engineer" of the data collection by modality is the trial-and-error of natural selection over eons of geologic time. Georg Cantor's conceptual realization (set theory) which is the lynch-pin of empirical mathematics, was anticipated by evolution and natural selection. It is amusing to recall that, as Einstein initially resented quantum theory, set-theory was resented by eminent mathematicians when first published. Poincaré, who remains a giant in mathematics declared set-theory to be a disease that he hoped to see disappear.

The topographic, macroscopic and microscopic organization of the neocortex into symbolic data sets is the insight allowing the deduction of how data are processed in the neocortex: 1. All data about the world always and only concerns the surface of physical matter and some of its properties, be it surfaces in contact with skin, light, or sound emitted or reflected from non-juxtaposed surfaces, or molecules emitted from surfaces. 2. Regardless of the peripheral detecting device (for light only, sound only, apposed surfaces only, etc.) all devices relay their activations in the form of trains of bioelectric potentials. 3. Bioelectric potentials from discrete detector modalities are received in topographically demarcated and distinct cortical regions which are ipso facto data sets. 4. Three of the six neuronal data sets are internally organized in fixed, homuncular patterns: somesthesia, kinesthesia, and the motor strip. Thus, potentials from stimulated cheek skin always activate receptor neurons in the postrolandic parietal convexity behind those from skin of the hand; signals commanding variations of foot muscles always depart that portion of the motor strip at the bottom and in front of the Rolandic fissures (mesial posterior frontal cortex). Raw data consists of variations of cortical receptor or motor control neurons. The latter are in fact also receptor neurons—but not of sensory data. Rather, they are tantamount to rheostats, activated by "I" or "auto." Raw data always arrives in the sensory receptor areas as activations of neurons in those areas. Data always concerns surfaces of body or non-body items. Neuronal circuits must submit all incoming data to temporo-spatial, associative, averaging and probabilistic analysis. First-order products of analysis constitute first orders of awareness. In humans these are "touch," "smell," "taste," "hearing," and "sight." Additional neuronal-circuit processing involving cross-referencing and associational logic will, if performed, produce perceptions, ideas and verbal intellect. Thus, variations in the states of cortical neurons are noted, remembered, filed in symbolic registries representing discrete functional modalities and these last—due to perpetual repetition of particular sequences *in time* (always reproducible within and between registered modalities)—undergo averaging and cross-referencing analysis. Physically, neuronal cross-references and associations are simply synapses between symbolic neuronal-circuit variables. For example, the neuronal cross-reference for English "house" and Hebrew "bayit" (linguistic symbols for the same item) must be synapses linking a neuronal symbol for house, and another for bayit, which are separated in cerebral space. Similarly for associations: the neuronal arrangement symbolizing barking sounds may be synaptically linked to the neuronal visual symbolic arrangement for dogs, separated from it in neocortical space. Such synapses constitute physical links between empirically verifiable phenoma. Synaptic associations may also form in cases of faulty or defective empirical verification, as when the first time one registers barking no dog is visible and a distant bird is seen to open and close its beak, the bird-sound being drowned out by the barking. A tentative association-synapse forms between "bark" and "bird." But since many phenomena recur in the world, one eventually registers that birds chirp and eventually dogs are seen while barking, so the neuronal-circuit averaging mechanism revises the physical synaptic links connecting "dog" to "bark" and "bird" to "chirp" while dissolving "bird"—"bark."

The neopallial nervous *system* comprises peripheral tissues constituting organs specialized to detect finite and limited bands in spectra of matter and energy; a central element (the neocortex) which receives and processes potentials from triggered detectors and relays potentials to the third constituent of the system: "voluntary" muscles under the detectors and which the neocortex must learn to stimulate so as to interact with and survive in the environment. The system was produced by natural selection and evolution. Human neurons monitor and survive the environment by mastering only five alarm systems: our five "senses." Each alarm is routed to a distinct area of the necortex, resulting in topographic separation (initially only—at the points of arrival of signals) into five sensory data sets. Processing of potentials by circuits downstream of each receptor cortex yields progressive spatial and functional convergence of data modalities via association tracts culminating in functional fusion of sensory data which is an input of "I's" localized in the neocortex. Elaborating awareness requires deducing the functional relationship between data sets followed by determination of their individual functional significance. The degree, quality, and orders of complexity of awareness and ultimately of mind depend on the qualitative and quantitative complexity of the total nervous *system* and the degree of integration of its parts. To discover the functional significance of potentials causing variations in cortical receptor neurons, brains must deduce that variations are signals and then deduce in a precise logical order what peripheral organ was triggered. The next step is to plot the temporal shape and dimensions of the body surface (skin). Success allows brains to explore and categorize some of the world surrounding the body. Phylogenetically and in all babies—regardless of species—development of multicellular long-range sensations (so-called) is contingent on and necessarily consecutive to formation of the concept of the body surface which depends on the "direct" sensation of "touch." Brains are in part biological computers (they are more than that but it is their indisputable computer persona that is relevant to our discussion). Their ultimate computer product, as far as we can tell, is the human mind. They were "engineered" (and were fine-tuned by natural selection for) to monitor the macro world and survive in it. To do so successfully they must fit all environmental phenomena in one of the three survival categories: dangerous, beneficial, and indifferent. This breakdown mandates just three general kinds of response: neutralize dangers, exploit the beneficial, do not offend the indifferent. Unlike man-made computers where possibilities of input and output are constrained by previous human programming, the biologic computers that brains are have self-learning and self-improvement capabilities of lesser or greater extent, depending on the "design" of the individual brain and the nervous system it forms part of. This obtains because brains are functionally and obligatorily linked in a closed loop with "somesthetic" (i.e. tactile) inputs contingent on non-body stimulations at any given moment, and outputs (voluntary muscles activations) responding to one of the three survival imperatives. In order to promote survival in the macro world, neurons which are synaptically and functionally integrated as circuits have no other option but to view time/space as the invariable matrix of the universe and matter/energy as reliefs on this matrix. This obtains because neurons don't know cytology (hence themselves), nor physics and mathematics (although neuronal circuits *apply* physics and mathematic symbolically to arrive at symbolic deductions. It is not necessary to know chemistry to make fire). Because matter/energy are crucial to survival, it suffices to register that they are relatively concentrated or dilute and thus detectable at and above quantitative and qualitative thresholds of concentration. Natural selection provides animal species with a small number of organic sensing devices, each primed for triggering at threshold concentrations of matter/energy, but not below said thresholds. That is why human vision excludes infrared and ultraviolet (detectable by members of some species) while our auditory range excludes "high" and "low" sound frequencies which are detectable by dogs and elephants, and our ability to monitor odors is at least two orders of magnitude less than pigs'. To survive it suffices to register three categories of unit concentrations of matter/energy: solid, liquid, and gas, and two functional states: living or inanimate. Brains qua computers are the central element in an input-output system for identifying and solving survival problems. They are therefore more or less adept at self-tuning to better promote survival. Brains are obligated biologic computers. Single or persistent failures to solve survival dilemmas inevitably lead to death. Mathematically and materially it is not possible to provide advance data (or any at all) in advance, nor "all" formulae and equations for solving all challenges the world may pose. But survival does not require total understanding of the universe and its individual components. It is enough to localize and monitor those ingredients of the world bearing on survival and to deal with them appropriately regardless of whether one understand their ins and outs. For example, most living beings cannot discover the physico-chemical bases of combustion yet they usually react appropriately to fire, trying to avoid burning themselves and sometimes (the case of some birds) stalking behind fire to eat its victims.

Let signals from skin bear a (for neurons) symbol: "S," and from stimulated muscles, "Mf" for flexor, and "Me" for extensor muscles coupled with the flexors. Roughly the same receptor neurons receive signals from foot skin (depending on the area of stimulation) and muscles (depending on degree and ratio of flexor/extensor muscle variation), each time the same skin surface area is stimulated and underlying, paired flexors/extensors caused to undergo reflex variations and similarly for leg skin-leg muscles variations in cephalic progression until the skin and muscles of the scalp.

Then: since the computer role of the new brains requires them to receive signals, they must sort these signals into as-yet-unknown categories. Let signals from (skin-of-foot-followed-by-subsequently-varying-foot-muscles) be symbolized: "Sx-Mx," and those from (skin-of-leg-followed-by-subsequently-varying-leg-muscles) by "Sy-My" and so on upward to scalp skin-muscles. After the brain plots the contours of foot, leg, and thigh these become, respectively, "Sf-Mf," "Sl-Ml," and "St-Mt" etc. all the way to the scalp ("Ss-Ms"). Note that the triple retreat reflex consists of sequential variations of muscles from those furthest from the head to those closer to it—a precise, tail-to-head reconstruction of actual external anatomy. In the lower extremities the progression is (immutably): foot, leg, thigh. In the upper extremities (viz: stimulation of skin of thumb) it is: extension of all fingers, extension of hand on forearm, forearm on arm, and abduction of arm from shoulder. The order of reflex contraction is always the same. Immutability and reproducibility, then: essential for any measurement.

We know from the work of anatomists and physiologists that many brain-body interactions are crossed. Tactile signals of one side of the body are relayed to the controlateral cerebral hemisphere; we monitor the world on the right of our midline with our left occipital lobe; voluntary muscle activity to one side of our midline is ordered from the opposite cerebral hemisphere. Crossed brain-body interactions are not absolute. Both inner ears send signals to each posterior temporal lobe, and the frontalis muscle in the forehead is stimulated by both motor strips. Also, infants who undergo resection of a cerebral hemisphere before crossed brain-body tracts become fixed, control both sides of the body with the remaining hemisphere and monitor the world on either side of the midline with it alone. After crossed pathways become fixed, damage in part or all of one hemisphere impairs or prevents control of muscles in the controlateral body and/or impairs or blocks "sensations" from the controlateral body. This is one aspect of the provable phenomenology of body-brain interactions. Our purpose is to show how awareness is produced by using established macroscopic, microscopic, and physiologic facts concerning brains and bodies. To that end, it suffices to note that clearly-demarcated macroscopic cortical sensory receptor areas are functional data sets as is each motor strip. "I" must learn which motor strip neurons to stimulate to effect precise muscle variations. Newborn brains enter the world equipped with flexor/extensor muscles registries passively formed in-utero/ovo (whose meaning remains to discover), immediate recall circuits, and rudimentary "I's." Their challenge is to "make sense" of variations in the somesthetic (tactile), kinesthetic (flexor/extensor muscle "sensation") and motor strip areas so as to form a reference point for variations in the remaining "sensory" cortices – while *every* receptor region constantly receives potentials from "sense organs" which were inactive prenatally. Because they are functional data sets, the cortical receptor regions are analogous to man-made electronic consoles, each varying only for one specific input. This fact makes it necessary that neuronal circuits establish relationships between "consoles" (data sets) sans awareness of the existence of said "consoles" and without the possibility of observing them. Another helpful console-cortex analogy is that each console contains a finite number of pixels. Individual pixels are, or are not electronically active, each pixel of each console being activated only by a specific constituent of the input which is itself specific only for that console, while cortical receptor regions are composed of neurons bearing a stereotypical relation to individual components of the input to each region, so that specific neurons in a region always and only are or are not active when their discrete input is or is not triggered. Individual pixels or neurons are therefore either "on" or "off" regardless whether what activates them concerns pressure/texture/temperature, sound, light etc. Biologic evolution fine-tuned by natural selection made the neocortex a physical embodiment of set theory to facilitate the elaboration of consciousness and thus enhance survivability. Georg Cantor, unversed in Neurology, couldn't know this despite discovering set theory, nor (to my knowledge) has anyone who has not authored or read or been influenced by this manuscript or its predecessor.

Newborns enter the world with neocortices functionally segregated into data sets ("consoles") receiving potentials from sense organs triggered by matter apposed to skin (including body parts in juxtaposition), light and sound from items *not* contacting eyes or ears, etc. Data sets responding to triggering of skin and muscles are the somesthetic cortices (right, left, primary, secondary and tertiary), the sensory flexor/extensor muscle variation cortices (flexor and extensor muscle couples vary inversely) triggered by the polysynaptic reflex and later by the neocortex), a joint-position cortex (one right, one left and allowing determination of spatial location of limb segments) and the bilateral motor strips and their supplementary areas, the strips being triggered within the brain by "I" or "auto." The muscles-variation cortices literally reflect the numbers of motor units contracting in a muscle (the higher the number, the greater the force of contraction) and the proportionately inverse relaxation of motor units in the coupled antagonist muscle. In the poly-synaptic reflex (a frequent phenomenon of early life) signals arrive to the cortical "consoles" in the order: somesthetic, kinesthetic (flexor/extensor muscle variations) and proprioceptive (joint position, which varies when flexor/extensor variations are sufficient to displace segments of limbs). Let us summarize the sequence as: 1, 2, 3. But if muscle couples are made to vary by *cerebral* command and two skin areas are not apposed nor a limb brought to "touch" a non-body surface, "I" records the cerebral sequence: 0, 2, 3 if muscle contraction caused movement of a limb around joint(s), or simply "0," 2 (we are aware of flexing or relaxing our muscles. Therefore "I" or IA – meaning interoactivation – is at the same time the time-zero of the sequence, and the memory of its initiation). If interoactivation brings portions of skin into apposition, the neocortical sequence becomes: "0"-2-3-(1-1) and if skin contacts non-body surfaces it becomes: "0"-2-3-1. Learning involves, in the first instance, deducing that variations occurring in the cortical "consoles" are *determined* by variations of sensors at the body surface *even when the trigger is a cerebral command to skeletal muscles.* Even when force of contraction of muscles to cerebral command is too weak to displace a limb segment around its joint, the feedback sensory flexion/extension variation was generated from the *muscles* and hence at the periphery. Integrating data sets consists in forming synapses between them. The synaptic linking is guided by logic circuits, themselves contingent internally and externally on synaptic formation. Therefore, consciousness must be built in the following order:

1. Interpolation (discovering the body surface).
   a. Discovering the functional relations between data sets.
   b. Discovering the functional significance of data.

c. Dscovering the functional axes of the body (polar coordination).
d. apping the body surface (curve fitting).

2. Extrapolation: discovery of the non-body world by reference to the polar coordinates (axes) of the body.

The brain considers the body party of "I" although some of it can be sacrificed to safeguard "I." Brains can tolerate losses of body parts if the parts are not crucial for staying alive, and if blood loss, shock and infection are not excessive.

Brains are central components of the neocortical nervous system tetrad. The other components are peripheral sense organs, input tracts linking them to the neocortex, and the motor output tracts linking the motor strips to muscles. The system functions by monitoring the macro world and commanding responses to it. Histologically and functionally human brains have three parts: paleopallium, phylogenetically the oldest, composed of particular cells in the rhinencephalon – olfactory bulb, tract, tubercle and striae, the anterior olfactory nucleus, parts of the amygdaloid complex, and parts of the pre-pyriform cortex; archepallium, next in appearance phyolgenetically, consisting of the hippocampus, dentate and fasciolar gyri, and indusium griseum (supracallosal gyrus); neopallium, phlogenetically the youngest and represented by the most superficial brain layer, the neocortex. The neocortex has six cell layers, the paleo and archepallia less. The neocortex and its six cell layers is what is conventionally termed the thinking brain. In this book, paleo and archepallia are functionally labeled the autonomic, or non-thinking brain. It is always active, monitoring and regulating respiration, heart rate, blood pressure, muscle tone, blood content of 02, C02, glucose, pH etc whether we are awake or asleep. The thinking brain actively deals with the macro world only while we are awake. It is inactive in sleep and coma, when the autonomic brain ensures homeostasis as best it can. The autonomic brain antedates the "thinking" brain phylogenetically and embryologically. It regulates the delivery of fuel and oxygen to the neocortex. It physically provides the first bioelectric stimuli to neocortical neurons and ipso facto their first lessons or instructions. Now, let us recall the rationale for multicellularity. Both uni and multicellular beings want to stay alive and intact. Individual protozoans have poor odds of success at this if their only defense against microscopic hazards is the lock and key mechanism of their cell membrane. This is so inadequate that at least two solutions have evolved. One is rapid reduplication. It takes time to penetrate cell membranes. The likelihood of encountering agents devoted to harmful cell penetration is time-related. Therefore survival of protozoan colonies (but not necessarily their individual members) is enhanced by reduplicating faster than the average time between lethal encounters. Some bacteria and protozoa reproduce every half-hour, and for all I know there might be faster reproduction rates. The second solution, culminating in the human mind, is multicellularity. Properly engineered, multicellularity allows neurons (which have no "senses") to survive repeated encounters with hazardous agents by interposing a host of shields between themselves and hazardous agents: bone, blood vessels, skin, the internal organs, the immune system. Multiple encounters with lethal microscopic agents are deferred. The raw nature confronting neurons is the macroscopic universe, and the body is a puppet propped by neurons to deal with it. Their survival odds are apparently acceptable vis a vis the macro, because the puppet often survives injuries or damage which would be fatal to naked neurons. With all the dangers of the macro world, the fact that you are reading this means that your neurons have lived considerably longer than is usual for individual one-celled animals. And longevity permits formation of relatively voluminous data banks concerning dangerous and benevolent items, their detection and suitable responses to them. One-celled organisms have two options for direct assessment of surrounding matter: contact of cell membrane with matter of the same order of magnitude, and molecular stimulation of the cell membrane. Molecule-membrane interaction is direct in protozoa, but indirect in metazoans since the cells registering the fact of molecular stimulation of end-organs (i.e. of taste buds and cells in the nasal mucosa) are not the cells stimulated by the molecules, but cerebral neurons (which are only *signaled* that molecules are titillating nose or palate). So although "smell" and "taste" are considered long-range "sensations," they are (for cerebral neurons) actually symbolic metaphors for the second kind of protozoan direct contact with a cell's surrounding matter – molecular as opposed to mechanical (pressure, texture being mechanical and simply a function of the size of the stimulus). Unicellular phototropism is a long-range detection mechanism for which the multicellular analogue is "vision." Protozoa thus have two means of direct detection, chemical and tactile, while metazoa have none. All detection by neurons is indirect (non-neuronal cells are triggered by macroscopic matter/energy, signaling the fact of being triggered to the neocortex by bioelectric discharges). The fact is that for *neurons* all detection of events at the body surface (and within the body as well) is *actually* indirect and long-range, but mechanical contact of matter with skin, or chemical contact with nose and palate are *equated* with the direct stimulation of protozoan cell membranes, sight (the analogue of phototropism) remains a long-range modality, and hearing (the analogue of vibrations directly contacting cell membranes) is symbolically transformed in metazoans into a long-range "sensory" modality. The skin of the feet of six footers is about six feet removed from their brain, but their neocortex has symbolically rendered skin the functional equivalent of protozoan cell membranes. Skin is held to be the demarcation between "me" and non-me while the reality is that "I" is a functional integration of neocortical inputs and outputs, physically confined in the neocortex, and the part of "my" envelope called "scalp" (the section of skin closest to "me") is centimeters distant from any neuronal cell membrane (actually close to one foot, since signals from the scalp have to transit in the second and third cervical spinal cord segments – roughly six inches from the crown – and then ascend almost as far to reach the somesthetic cortex). In tall people, skin of the feet is meters distant from "I." What "I" calls "direct" contact with macro matter is direct only because of the equation "skin = cell membrane." This equation is a requirement of multicellular symbolism. It is realized by a conceptual sleight of hand, for this reason: By intention, neurons' location precludes their detection of matter either proximately or at long range (that's the purpose of multicellularity), be they in invertebrate heads (cephalopods, spiders et al) or in vertebrate ones (fish, amphibia and "up"). Therefore, cells other than neurons do the detecting, those symbolizing contact with cell membranes (i.e. direct contact) being mechanoreceptors embedded in skin and those symbolizing long-range clumped in retinae, cochleae, taste buds, nasal mucosa, Jacobson's organs (snakes' means of sensing animal heat) lateral line (fishes' organs sensing bioelectricity) and similarly for echolocation in bats and cetaceans. As amoebic cell membranes form pseudopods, their analogue in various metazoa are locally constituted into appendages serving to displace the animal or to seize things (arms bearing hands, legs, invertebrates' tentacles, elephant trunks etc). For functioning in detection mode, they are supplemented by mechanoreceptors and tracts transmitting potentials from them to the neocortex allowing it to establish that matter was, or not, encountered. It follows that for brain cells, any device (i.e. organ) activated by matter/energy is a detector provided something is relayed to the processing unit (brain) whose logic functions (cell circuits) will eventually deduce that the something relayed signifies activation of the organ. Once brains establish that reception of signals means organs were triggered, then variations in the sensory receptor areas signify: detection of pressure, molecules, light and sound. Variations of neocortical receptor neurons are not actually light, sound, pressure etc. But brains assign specific symbolic values to each "sensory" modality, said value standing for the physical phenomenon triggering each type of peripheral "sense" organ. Consequently, A: Activation of peripheral organs becomes both necessary and sufficient to posit that a factor (x) has triggered the peripheral organ. B: Activation caused the organ to undergo a chemical, mechanical or electrical variation. C: The variation was electrically propagated to the brain (brains can deduce only that organs were triggered and signals relayed, not the physical forms of variation and propagation). D: Variations of neurons in the receptor areas constitute signal-reception and therefore constitute data, even though the physical forms of activation and relay are different from the physical forms of agents triggering peripheral detectors. E: The first "assignment" of biologic computers (brains), unlike man-made ones, is to deduce that variations of cortical receptor neurons are signals, and then what is being signaled. Therefore, brains can form only symbolic equivalents of contents of the physical world. The symbols are spatial/dynamic constructs of neocortical neurons. They result from analysis, by neocortical neuronal logic circuits, of detections of non-body items by specialized biologic detectors composed of cells which are *not* neurons, separated from the neocortex by distances which are enormous at the microscopic scale. In other words, no data concerns the cell membranes of neurons. All data is therefore indirect. The cell membrane is its boundary between self and non-self, but neurons of multicellular organisms are required to equate the skin (which is the boundary of multicellular organisms but not of their neurons, between organism and non-organism) with their cell membranes. As "I" is a fusion of neocortical inputs and outputs, so the skin is a conceptual metaphor for "I" of the demarcation between the multicellular *organism* and non-"I," a metaphor "I" must formulate and believe in order to make "sense" of signals by non-neurons located very far from them in microscopic terms, and also in order to efficiently command muscles under the metaphoric "I"-"non-I" boundary so as to maneuver the multicellular organism in a manner best calculated to ensure neocortical survival and comfort. The multicellular collective must be viewed as "I" *by* "I" so that "I" can best assure its survival by making use of what the collective tells "I" about the macro world and maneuver the collective accordingly. View these logical requirements, organs are detection devices not because of their powers of resolution ("grain") but by virtue of always transmitting signals when triggered. All detectors – biologic and manufactured – have limits of resolution – the "visible" spectrum; sound (hearing) frequency band, smell/taste thresholds (thresholds of molecular concentration) etc. Powers of resolution and thresholds vary between species and among individual species members. The practical consequence of the foregoing is that detection by biologic sensors cannot possibly identify everything in the macro world. Humans don't "see" infrared and ultraviolet, "hear" high/low frequency sounds etc. Nor can discrete macro items be totally known through sensations alone. We do not see the cells we are made of, bacteria on our skin, or the shape of the Earth we live on. Neuronal conclusions from processed sensory data are necessarily idiosyncratic – the ground seems flat while in reality planets are spherical. Another barrier to omniscience is that no matter the longevity, no lifetime is sufficiently long to encounter all the contents of the macro universe. And, organisms live in ecological niches – fish cannot exist in alpine non-aqueous habitats. But survival does not need the impossible (total detection), merely adequate detection. Any device activated by matter will serve for detection provided cerebral circuits will process signals that it is triggered and discover the triggering phenomenon. Neocortical neuronal circuits downstream of the receptor cortices process and analyze variations of receptor neurons so as to symbolically reconstruct finite aspects of the macro world. To do so they need chronologic or spatial means for measuring – that is, for comparing – events in the cortical receptor areas. The brain's physical organization, cytology and physiology determine what form of comparison (temporal or spatial) is possible. The immobility of neurons and their separation in cerebral space allow some neurons organized in circuits to compare the *chronologic* relations of neuronal variations in two or more regions of space (whether events are simultaneous or non-simultaneous) because of the computer attributes of the brain. The spatial distinctness of intracerebral events is *not* measurable by any functional structures in the brain. Given that brains are, in part, biologic computers, I venture that their processing of data is binary. More significantly, deductions are arrived at by applying binary *logic*: something is, or is not; things are, or are not. Because of cerebral cytology and physiology, brains experience time as one-dimensional and use time-based units of measurement to compare the spatial dimensions of items in the macro world. Acquiring the concept of the relative proportions of the body surface results from differences in times of arrival of muscles variably distant from "I' when "I" stimulates two or more muscles simultaneously. Variable distances and equal conduction velocities result in variable arrivals in time of signals from stimulated muscles. Recall that foot muscles are under the skin of the feet, hand muscles under the skin of the hands etc. The relative dimensions of hands and feet are found by comparing differences in arrival times of signals from hand and foot muscles which were ordered to vary simultaneously by "I." Resultant concepts of size are applied to measuring the height of horses in "hands" and small linear ground distances in "feet." *Because* time-based units are used to define macroscopic spatial dimensions, brains experience time as one-dimensional, space as three-dimensional, "dimension" referring to the quantity of numbers necessary to define something – i.e., space, having length, breadth and width is three-dimensional while weight and voltage, like time, appear one-dimensional. Other examples of using time to measure space: locations are 20 minutes' brisk walk away, or three days by sailboat… Again: at the neuronal cell-circuit level units of time are used to discover and measure space, which is the reason we "feel" time as one, and space as three-dimensional.

After plotting the shape and dimensions of the body surface, and in order to continue with the discovery and itemization of the non-body world, neocortical neuronal-circuit operations *must* be subsumed to the following principles of logic:

1. All deductions are based on processed data.
2. All measurement consists of comparing material items with an arbitrary unit of measurement.
3. All units of measurement are arbitrary.
4. Therefore arbitrary units of measurement are fixed variables in a binary logic system. If an arbitrary unit be designated "U," then all other material items are "Non-U." "U" and "Non-U" can be logically manipulated a la Boolean "and," "or" and "not:"
   a. U and Non-U
   b. U or Non-U
   c. U not Non-U

   The logical corollary of this is "Therefore" and thus: U *therefore* Non-U.
5. Since Non-U is a logical *hypothesis*, neuronal circuits stretch a relative truth into an absolute one – e.g., "my" hand *is* "me" and a table is "non-me." In reality, given adequate medical care, neurons can survive destruction of both table and hand. But they must *logically* form a "U"-"Non-U" hypothesis about the skin of the multicellular collective and all other ingredients of the macroscopic universe. This logical necessity arises because neurons need an arbitrary unit with which to compare all

material items of the macro universe. That "Unit" can only be the body – or rather, the outer boundary of the multicellular collective and specifically its envelope, the skin which is a metaphor for a cell membrane.

6. The body is the brain's arbitrary unit for measuring all items of the macro world. Therefore, for processing according to binary logic, neurons consider the body envelope (skin) "B," and everything outside "Non-B." "Non-B" is, then, by definition, all non-body matter/energy, while ("B" and "B") is the neocortical *deduction*: body surface (skin), conventionally termed "somesthesia" (tact) and ("B" not "B") is awareness *that* the envelope or a portion of the envelope is in non-body space and not contacting anything.
7. If neuronal analysis concerning individual non-body items stops at (therefore non-b), the items are merely identified as outside the envelope. If logical processing is pursued so as to deduce (non-B therefore X), a higher order of cognition is expressed. A simple "non-B" is a primary deduction corresponding to the conventional meaning of "sensation," while "Non-B therefore X" is that order of awareness understood by the word "perception."

For the neocortex, "I" is the arbitrary center-point from which the shape and relative dimensions of the body-envelope is plotted using units of time measurement (brain-muscle-brain latencies). All measurement *must* depart from an arbitrary reference-point, and the only such point available to the neocortex is "I." As "I" is the reference-point for measuring the body surface and calculating the relative proportions of segments of that surface (limbs, head, trunk, thorax, abdomen), so the body is the reference-point for judging the dimensions and relative proportions of non-body macro items. "I" serving as point of reference for plotting the body surface may be diagrammatically represented as in Figure 7. Here, all vectors from "I" are centrifugal and correspond to brain-muscle-brain time latencies: the distances of muscles from the neocortex in time.

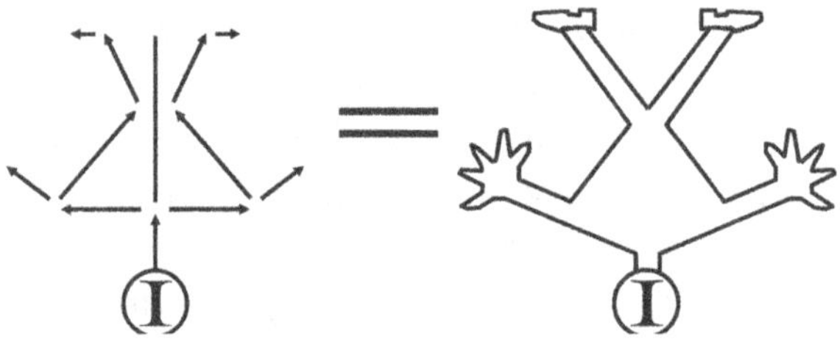

Figure 7: Plotting the Body Surface using Brain-Muscle-Brain Chronologic Latencies to Measure Linear Distances, with "I" as Central Reference-Point.

Here, vectors are centrifugal (away from "I') because brains establish how far muscles are removed in time. They cannot take into account the round-trip nature of brain-muscle-brain exchanges.

Muscle cells specialize in lengthening or shortening, endocrine cells in producing and secreting hormones, and neurons in varying electric state and propagating and receiving bioelectric potentials which can cause variations of electric states. Neurons specialize in receiving and transmitting bioelectricity. Since all aspects of the macro world are signaled to brains in the form of bioelectric potentials; since neurons can only receive and transmit potentials and potentials received in the neocortex are differentiated into sundry "sensations": then differentiation must occur downstream of neocortical receptor neurons via symbolic logical processing expressible by formulae. The hierarchical place of a formula in the ascending logic cascade defines the material structures of the symbolic items "sensations," "perceptions" and "ideas."

We have mentioned segmental mono-and-polysynaptic reflex arcs. A reflex is an immutable sequence of events proceeding in a stereotypical order following adequate stimulation. Since the only relationship of neurons with the macro world is arrivals of bioelectric potentials in some cortices (causing receptor neurons to vary in electrical state) and relay of potentials from other neocortical neurons to muscles, then there must be some immutable and stereotypical combination of somesthetic and kinesthetic potentials arriving in the somesthetic and kinesthetic (receptor) areas corresponding to polysynaptic reflexes, and a logic system composed of neuronal circuits for discovering the stereotypy, comparing times of arrival and concluding to the functional significance of same. The process is necessarily inductive (from specific to general) because the only links possible between neurons are synapses, and this applies, as well, to events in neocortical space involving two or more areas. Now, in clinical Neurology latencies of conduction along peripheral nerves are routinely determined by nerve conduction studies. Normal latencies are in the thousandth of second range. For example, recording electrodes are taped to the ball of the thumb (containing mostly median-nerve innervated muscles) and the median nerve is stimulated through the skin at the wrist 8-cm from the recording electrode. Normal motor latencies are 3.8 thousandths second or faster. Sensory fibers of the same nerve normally relay potentials over a 14-cm distance at 3.2 milliseconds or faster. Commands from cortex to muscles must travel to a segmental spinal cord level and exit into a motor nerve to the muscle, while signals from responding flexor/extensor antagonist muscle couples return to the cortex in a roughly reverse manner. Thus, commands from cortex to human lip or forehead muscles proceed from cortex to cervical spinal cord in the pyramidal tract, and to the muscles in the facial (7th cranial) nerve. The muscle response returns in a sensory nerve (5th cranial or trigeminal) to the cord, then in a sensory tract from the pons to the thalamus and finally to the kinesthetic cortex. In average-sized men the round trip is between 0.5 – 0.6 meter. In six footers (1.8 meter), the brain-foot distance is roughly 1.8 meter and the return signal from muscles identical, so the linear distance is 3.6-m or approximately 11.8-ft. Now, peripheral nerves are bundles of nerve fibers ranging from 0.5 to 22 micrometers in diameter. One micrometer ("micron") is one millionths meter or one thousandths millimeter. Satellites called Schwann cells envelope each fiber in a thin cytoplasmic tube covered by the neurilemma (sheath of Schwann). Within the neurilemma, Schwann cells further wrap larger fibers in a multilayered insulating membrane, the myelin sheath. In the brain and spinal cord cells called oligodendrocytes encase nerve fibers in myelin. Adjacent segments join at so-called Nodes of Ranvier. Bioelectric potentials travel in peripheral nerve tracts from one Node of Ranvier to the next ("saltatory conduction"). If memory serves, a red blood cell is about 7 microns (0.007-mm) in diameter. 142.8 contiguously aligned red cells equal one millimeter. If neurons are roughly the same diameter as red blood cells, a nerve bundle 22 microns long encased in myelin contains three neurons in alignment and signals traveling along the myelin sheath bypass every three neurons. The ulnar nerve's forearm segment has a conduction velocity in normals of roughly 50 meters/sec, or 164-ft/sec or 50,000-mm/sec, a fairly standard conduction velocity. Fifty thousand-mm contain 7,140,000 contiguously aligned red blood cells. There are no nodes of Ranvier in the receptor cortices, but although potentials cannot skip every three cells as in a 22-micron fiber bundle, it is difficult to see how conduction from one cortical neuron to another is measurable with current technology. Electric discharges by cells are followed by recovery ("refractory") periods, but the *relay* from a cell to its synaptic neighbor must be in the 50,000-mm/sec range and there is simply no way of placing electrodes in contiguous neurons to measure this. But since "brains" must "make sense" of variations of individual cortical neurons receiving potentials from the periphery, circuits downstream of the receptor neurons must be monitoring differences in activity of adjacent neurons. Saying this is impossible because such measurement is impossible with current technology is to overlook the fact that brains know that dogs are biting thousandths of a second after jaws clamp on ankles. If they did not, no one would ever escape further injury.

All signals received in the neocortex about the macro world concern surfaces: contact of body parts with each other or non-body surfaces, light reflecting from surfaces or sound and molecules emanating from surfaces. Neurons in several neocortical reception areas may vary simultaneously when peripheral organs are triggered by one or more environmental phenomena. Potentials received in somesthetic, visual, auditory, olfactory and gustatory cortices may concern same or different items. One might simultaneously see, touch, smell and hear a dog at the same time as one also hears a train whistle, smell roses in bloom and so on. Ability to hear simultaneous sounds is the first requirement for a musical conducting career. Brains must decide, in a first deductive step, that signals are being received, and, second, that they concern surfaces. That signals concern same or different items (i.e. touch-smell-sight-sound of dog and also train-whistle and lightening) is determined by synaptic associations between the various deductions. The division of the neocortex into spatially segregated sensory receptor regions subject to simultaneous variations and downstream processing and the option of forming synaptic links associating discrete prints-out of sensory data, renders brains the a protoplasmic equivalent of computers. Their "purpose" is ensuring survival in the macro world, while procreation is a joint goal of the autonomic brain and neocortex. And here, finally is the detailed, chronologic process brains must engage in to achieve their purpose.

Striated muscles signal their variations to the neocortex by relaying potentials in sensory fibers of mixed nerves. The latter join "sensory" nerve roots at the posterior segmental spinal cord level, signals entering the cord and continuing to, eventually, activate neurons in the kinesthetic (receptor) cortex which might be a "supplementary" somesthetic area. In healthy animals the muscle-to-cortex temporal latency is relatively constant. Cold slows conduction velocities, but equally in all nerves and central tracts, so differences due to distance are unchanged, and chronologic relations of muscles of different distance from the neocortex don't vary. The relative chronologic lengths of muscles unequally distant from the brain remain constant whether muscles very reflexly to skin stimulation or in response to neocortical commands. Cerebral commands to muscles are the only phenomena which can be initiated and verified by "I." Let interoactivation (IA) mean variation of striated muscles on cerebral command, and exteroactivation (EA) mean reflex variation via the polysynaptic reflex arc, which is signaled to the neocortex following triggering of cutaneous mechanoreceptors by non-body matter or by contact of two body parts. This reflex becomes inhibited with cerebral maturation, reappearing in pathologic states such as stroke, multiples sclerosis, brain tumors, and brain/spinal cord trauma. "Latency" is the time taken by a potential to traverse a fixed distance. In the laboratory, specific latencies for specific nerves are determined by placing electrodes in or over muscles and stimulating the nerves to the muscles at arbitrarily designated, fixed distances from the active electrode. Conduction velocities are determined by stimulating nerves close to the recording electrode and further away, measuring the distance between points stimulated, subtracting the shorter from the longer latency and dividing the result into the distance between stimulation points: $\text{Nerve Conduction Velocity} = \frac{\text{distance}}{\text{longer-shorter latency}}$. Brains cannot determine latencies in actual units of time nor, obviously, can they determine conduction velocities. But they *can* simultaneously interoactivate muscles variously distant from "I" and register the different feedback responses causing variations in the kinesthetic cortex. Signals from muscles closest to "I" (e.g. lip muscles) invariably precede those from more distant ones (e.g. hand or foot muscles). To forestall objections that the differences (which must be in the thousandths of second range) are too small for neuronal circuits to distinguish, we note again that if brains couldn't do so, we could never extract ankles form dogs' jaws to avoid additional injury – after all, signals from damaged tissues arrive in the brain thousandths of a second after damage occurred. So, brains cannot determine latencies in milliseconds, nor can (or need) they determine conduction velocities. But they can establish, through repeated IAs that responses from simultaneously activated lip, hand, and foot muscles always arrive in the order: lip-hand-foot. These are chronologic latencies, and their relationship to each other in cases of simultaneous IA is invariable. Since "I's" are reference points brains use to plot the universe, these chronologic latencies (lips closer than hands closer than feet and no "I" beyond) demarcate the relative proportions and configuration of "I's" surface or envelope. Note that the limits are those of muscles, not skin distant from "I." However, because muscles underlying skin can be maneuvered so that portions of skin (which contain mechanoreceptors) contact surfaces, it is *as if* muscles equal distance of skin (measured in chronologic latencies) from "I." From this it follows that for brains, "simultaneous" means two things: That if IA is simultaneous, then responses from stimulated muscles arrive either simultaneously or non-simultaneously – another case of binary logic. We have argued previously that brains must use the subtleties inherent in these temporal notions to hypothesize the existence of space.

It will be recalled that the state and strength of muscular contraction/relaxation is influenced both reflexly and by cerebral command. Reflex variations occur via the polysynaptic reflex arc when skin is contacted by non-body matter and also when two parts of the body come in contact. The only things "brains" can register, however, is that two variations occurred (in the neocortex) in quick succession: first, variations responding to signals from skin (brains must learn this), then variations due to signals from stimulated flexor/extensor muscles couples (also something brains must learn). The number of neurons varying in the somatotypically-organized "somesthetic" cortex is directly proportional to the surface area of (say) foot skin in contact with another surface. And, since we can command gradations of muscular contraction or relaxation, a finite number of neurons in the prerolandic "motor strip" must be stimulated by "I" to produce gradations of contraction/relaxation for every muscle subject to cerebral control. For example, if a muscle has a total of 15 motor units, then maximal variation on cerebral command requires that 15 motor strip neurons emit centrifugal potentials, one potential for each motor unit. If minimal force is desired, just two cortical neurons might be stimulated by "I." And since each muscle has a finite number of motor units, variations of finite numbers of neurons in the kinesthetic cortex – numbers directly proportional to number of motor units – indicate the contractile or relaxation variance of each muscle. If the total number of motor units be 15, then the maximal contraction causes variations of 15 neurons in the kinesthetic cortex, minimal contraction only one or two etc. Since muscles work as agonist-antagonist pairs, the variance of agonist contraction (quantified in the kinesthetic cortex by variation of a specific number of neurons) varies inversely with variance of cortical neurons stimulated by the antagonist muscle. For example, if agonist contraction translates to activation of seven neurons in the kinesthetic cortex, then antagonist relaxation translates to inactivation of seven kinesthetic cortex neurons linked to the antagonist. Intracerebral neuronal circuits downstream of the kinesthetic receptor neurons must monitor inverse variations of kinesthetic cortex agonist/antagonist signals beginning with the slight variations possible in ovo/utero. If this seems an enormous task, consider that the average human brain is estimated to contain around one hundred billion neurons. The reason for this large number now becomes clear. Withal, it is estimated that most people use only ten percent of their brain-capacity. So, in the polysynaptic reflex, triggering cutaneous mechanoreceptors results in two consecutive *intracerebral* events: first, variation of a number of neurons in the "somesthetic" homunculus proportional to the surface skin area whose mechanoreceptors were triggered; second, inverse variations of neurons in the kinesthetic cortex linked to reflex-activated flexor/extensor muscle couples underlying the stimulated skin area. These variations, absent major muscle trauma, change very slowly over a lifetime, and occur repeatedly every day. We do lose muscle bulk and therefore motor units as we age, but the loss is gradual. Either constant or periodic cerebral averaging must compensate for differences in numbers of cortical neuron variations over years or decades. Variations of specific agonist/antagonist couples have upper and lower limits which can be memorized – else why have one hundred billion neurons? The data base which is the launch pad of cerebral self-learning culminating in sentience – the raw material of the first neuronal circuit processing – is the passive in ovo /utero creation in embryos, of registries of inversely proportional agonist/antagonist muscle variations (which is a cipher for prenatal brains). At birth, bodies are mechanically extended by pelvic bones or by small openings in eggs. Signals from cutaneous mechanoreceptors triggered by contact with the maternal pelvic opening or breach in the egg-shell begin causing variations of neurons in the somesthetic cortex, following in short order by signals from relaxing flexor and passively contracting extensor muscles causing inverse variations of neurons in the kinesthetic cortex. This is when brains begin recording and memorizing sequential variations of inversely proportional paired phenomena. Each pair has a fixed location on a *scale* of chronologic latencies. Later, these inversely proportional variations occupying fixed positions on the chronologic latency scale, will be paired with another variable which is specific for each muscle couple: the variations of specific neurons of the somesthetic homunculus which precede reflex variations of specific kinesthetic cortex agonist/antagonist couples. Since animals are subject to gravity, some portions of skin always contact non-body matter. In early postnatal life before cerebral and spinal cord inhibitory mechanisms form, such contacts trigger reflex agonist/antagonist muscle variations and proportional variations of neocortical kinesthetic neurons. Eventually brains, which tabulate and store data (or why have 100,000,000,000 neurons) must hypothesize that since specific variables frequently precede inverse variations of variables occupying fixed positions on chronologic latency scales (a conclusion from data averaging) then often, somehow, the first variables cause the second. Symbolically, $\Delta Sx \rightarrow \frac{+\Delta F_y}{-\Delta E_z}$.

That is, specific somesthetic variables often precede (hence cause) inverse variations (variances in contraction or relaxation) of specific (and always the same) flexor/extensor muscle pairs. Of course, at this stage it is not known that “S” corresponds to tactile “sensation” while “F” and “E” are muscles – that’s what acquiring consciousness is all about! Finding this out requires associations via synaptic links concerning actual events at the body surface. These events are the triggering of mechanoreceptors in portions of juxtaposed skin. This is a recurrent and frequent daily event which must be memorized and placed in a neuronal registry. Here, two sets of somesthetic cortex variations are followed by two sets of kinesthetic cortex inversely proportional variations. But when non-body matter contacts skin triggering reflex muscle variations, there is only *one* cortical somesthetic variance followed by a succession of cephalad kinesthetic cortex inverse variations. Therefore, after brains form symbolic concepts of the organism's envelope (= body surface, = skin) by processing receptor cortex variations separated in time, juxtaposition of body parts logically leads to the deduction: *contact. The "sense" called "touch" is really the deduction: "contact."* This is a first-order deduction, and all such deductions concerning variations in the "sensory" receptor cortices are what we call "sensations." In the case of "touch," the logical steps must be the following:

Repeated juxtapositions of body parts must result in intracortical registries of specific tabulated juxtapositions. The posterior scalp cannot contact the throat, nor the tip of the nose one's buttock etc. Palm and fingers of the right hand can contact all of the anterior body but only limited areas of the back. There is a finite number of possible body part juxtapositions and so a finite registry of juxtaposed body parts. Infants eventually command their muscles well enough to displace portions of limbs bearing mechanoreceptors in skin and appose them to a finite percentage of the body surface. Triggered mechanoreceptors of the juxtaposed skin areas relay signals to the somesthetic cortex. Soon after, the kinesthetic flexor/extensor muscle cortex undergoes specific, inversely proportional variations due to potentials arriving from reflex-stimulated muscle pairs – a sequence of cortical events not initiated by "me." Since "I" deduces from cortical variations caused by peripheral joint-position sensors where "my" body parts are in space, it deduces that when signals from two skin areas occur almost simultaneously, the body parts emitting signals must be very close to each other. After enough occurrences, "close" is changed to: in contact. Somesthesia, then, signifies: "Contact!" not "touch." The act of voluntarily apposing mechanoreceptors in skin to surfaces is described by the verb "to touch" and we eventually substitute the act for the sensation, calling the sensation: "touch." But not all cases of contact are voluntary. Our envelope may be contacted despite our best efforts to avoid it. Here, we have not willed "touch" but experienced "contact!." Cerebral commands to appose body parts are preceded, and remembered as the cortical variation which precedes, subsequent variations in the somesthetic cortex – or, to be exact, remembered as preceding specific somesthetic variations; "I" never knows that the variations occur in the somesthetic cortex. The cerebral command to activate specific muscles is an IA. IA is understood to be something willed by "I," so it is "I" which commands apposition of body parts. But when skin is contacted by non-willed non-body items (we don't mean soap or eyeglasses deliberately apposed to skin) the neocortex registers somesthetic variations *not* preceded by IA. Therefore, the two justifications for the non-body hypothesis are, first that somesthetic variations involve just one rather than two portions of skin plotted to be in contact, and second, that the somesthetic variations are not preceded by IA. So here is how this plays out in the logic cascade:

A. Actual event: Apposition of a portion of skin with a non-body surface elicits reflex contraction of underlying muscles and withdrawal of a limb segment in immature animals.

Cortical events: Variations of a finite number of neurons in the somesthetic cortex followed immediately by inversely proportional variations of specific numbers of neurons in the kinesthetic cortex. Or, to be exact, specific somesthetic variations are followed by specific, inversely proportional kinesthetic events ("I" doesn't know the variations occur in separate spatial regions because it can't observe anything, and because it is a fusion of inputs. *Fusion cancels space*): $\Delta\, Sx \rightarrow \Delta \begin{smallmatrix} +F \\ -E \end{smallmatrix}$ i.e., somesthetic x variation are followed in time by inversely proportional F/E variations. Inference: x causes the F/E variations.

B. Actual event: A first variance of somesthetic receptor neurons receiving potentials from the thumb is followed by consecutive, inversely proportional variations in the kinesthetic cortex of specific numbers of neurons. These variations are themselves followed in time by variations of specific numbers of neurons in two locations of the somesthetic cortex (the fusion of inputs called "I" registers only that two somesthetic variations are occurring, not where they occur not that it is neurons that vary). Suppose non-body matter contacted skin of dorsal thumb producing a flexion reflex: thumb flexes on palm, wrist on forearm, forearm on arm and arm abducts on shoulder, so thumb contacts chin. "I" registers:

$$\mathrm{ST} \rightarrow \Delta \frac{+\mathrm{FPB}}{-\mathrm{EP}} \rightarrow \Delta \frac{+\mathrm{FCU}}{-\mathrm{ECU}} \rightarrow \Delta \frac{+\mathrm{BT}}{-\mathrm{Tr}} \rightarrow \Delta\,\mathrm{SC} + \Delta\,\mathrm{St}$$

Read: somesthetic thumb variations followed by inverse kinesthetic variations of flexor policis brevis/extensor policis, then flexor carpi ulnaris/extensor carpi ulnaris then biceps brachii/triceps then simultaneous somesthetic chin-thumb variations.

Inference: An initial somesthetic variation caused a sequence of inversely proportional muscle variations culminating in two somesthetic variations.

C. Actual event: "I" commands muscles to cause displacement of body parts with three possible outcomes at the periphery:

1. The member contacts neither body nor non-body surfaces.
2. The member contacts a portion of skin causing two somesthetic variations.
3. The member contacts only non-body matter resulting in a single somesthetic variation after a series of inversely proportional kinesthetic variations.

Inferences:

1. "I" have caused a sequence of specific kinesthetic variations.
2. The sequence of kinesthetic variations "I" induced has caused two somesthetic variations in the same sector of space.
3. The sequence of variations "I" induced has caused a somesthetic variation – the reverse of occasions when somesthetic variations precede kinesthetic ones.

Therefore, the functional significance of somesthesia ("S") is that there has been contact of part of "my" envelope (skin) with a "me" or with a "non-I" surface. And since gravity ensures that some of "my" envelope (skin) is always relaying signals, then the envelope always maintains partial contact with parts of itself or with non-"I." Since some body segments never contact some others (nipples and heels; earlobes and calves) the envelope is at least partly rigid and has geometric contours which are discoverable by analysis of chronologic latencies. The configuration of the envelope (body surface) is therefore plotted and consigned to memory. Since we deduce when body parts are apposed (and this is *only* a *deduction*) it follows that when body parts signal "contact" but not with apposed body parts, the surface contacted is non-body. The universe therefore has non-me ingredients. Their dimensions (we are speaking of the macro world) will be assessed relative to the plotted dimensions of "my" envelope or segments thereof (feet and hands, for example).

It is only if and after brains actively make the preceding logical deductions that they can make additional deductions which allow them to reason out the functional significance of each non-contact sensory modality. What makes this possible is synaptic cross-indexing or cross referencing of variations occurring simultaneously for two or more "sensory" modalities (somesthetic-visual, somesthetic auditory, somesthetic-visual-auditory olfactory etc.) It is a fact that brains receive, analyze, and can respond to multiple, concurrent sensory (i.e.: data) inputs. Thus, when the position of the thumb is plotted relative to the body surface, eyelids are open, there is light, and the six extraocular muscles of each eye (which are voluntary muscles) conjugately orient the retinae in the direction of the thumb, at least some non-somesthetic signals (remember that biologic computer logic is binary) must concern the thumb. At this point, a detour is in order. It explains why consciousness must develop in precisely the sensory order I propose and why attempts to understand consciousness by research on visual "sensation" alone are futile. Many researchers confine themselves to the visual system believing this to be the optimal means of explaining what sentience is and how it forms. Readers so inclined may read the rationale in an article of DNA laureate Sir Francis Crick in the September, 1979 Scientific American or in a review of his book, "The Incredible Hypothesis," in the February, 1994 issue of OMNI magazine. Believers of this tactic publish articles making claims like the following:

"In advanced animals, most categories are learned. Monkeys can learn to categorize stimuli as animal or non-animal ... food or non-food... tree or non-tree... fish or non-fish ... and by ordinal number... The neural correlates of such perceptual categories might be found in brain areas that process visual form. The inferior temporal (IT) and prefrontal (PF) cortices are likely candidates; their neurons are sensitive to form ... and they are important for a wide range of visual behaviors ..." [4]

Now, it is established that the "primary" visual cortex is the occipital lobe area called the "striate" cortex or "area 17." There can be no question that variations (i.e. signals) in area 17 must be cross-referenced, via synaptic association tracts, with previously formed concepts stored in data banks elsewhere in the neocortex. Vision is a long-range "sensation" (remember that "sensations" are merely neuronal *deductions*). If eyelids are shut (something we can control and be conscious of) retinal cells cannot be triggered by light. If objects occlude the eyeballs, rods and cones can't register light. Ergo, contact of eyeballs (containing the cells which are triggered by light) with opaque objects precludes any visual detection whatsoever, and formation of visual concepts. The luminous aspects of material things can only acquire meaning after there has been active, self-taught acquisition of concepts of the tactile character of the corporal envelope and sundry, frequently encountered environmental items. Let us recall the basis of learning: new concepts are built on previously acquired ones. Evolution and embryology have contrived to require that the first awareness of

4. "Categorical Representation Of Visual Stimuli In The Primate Prefrontal Cortex," Freedman et al, Science magazine, Jan. 12, 2001

macroscopic phenomena is of animals' corporal envelope, their skin (animals with exoskeletons are born with the future rigid parts unhardened, so one assumes that they bear mechanoreceptors which are triggered before hardening is completed). Let us emphasize once again that skin isn't really neurons' envelope (they have cell membranes), but functionally skin is the multicellular animal's analog of one-celled animals' cell membrane which is their mechanical and chemical demarcation from one-celled microscopic items. Interfacing with the non-body macroscopic world obliges neocortical "I" to consider skin "its" envelope because it doesn't know it is a fusion of inputs and outputs of innumerable neurons having cell membranes and functioning in obligated intercollaboration. By stimulating variations of neurons in the motor strip (causing muscles to contract, displacing portions of limbs bearing mechanoreceptors in skin overlying the muscles) the neocortex activates a macroscopic "direct" brain-muscle-mechanoreceptor-brain feedback loop whenever brain-ordered muscle variations cause displaced limbs to contact surfaces. By contrast, there is no light, little sound, and few categories of molecules to "see," "hear," "smell" or "taste" in ovo/utero. Therefore, "somesthesia" (tactile "sensation") and the discovery of one's macroscopic envelope (the configuration of the body covered by skin) have got to be the first "sensory" modalities acquired. Once our external contour becomes known, signals from organs of long-range detection can start being processed by reference to the only thing as yet known – our body surface. To acquire meaning, the first visual signals must concern the envelope (body surface). Verifying the correctness of first visual deductions is done by self-palpation. For example, eyelids are open; there is light; proprioceptive signals inform the neocortex that the eyes are oriented toward the right thumb. The neocortex, having taught itself that somesthetic variations signify contact, is receiving sundry non-contact signals (i.e., is aware that sundry variations currently occurring – visual, auditory et al) are non-contact (but it doesn't yet know the meaning of any non-contact variations). It reasons (i.e. logic circuits do) that some of the non-contact signals concern the right thumb. Exploiting its new-found mastery of muscles combined with new-found ability to displace limbs via its control of muscles, it superimposes the left hand on the right thumb (or moves the right hand under the chin). Some of the non-contact variations (the visual ones concerning the thumb) cease. The variations that cease must concern the thumb. Certainty is established through repeated trials. Results are constant and reproducible. Data averaging circuits calculate that these variations are a non-contact aspect of the right thumb. The specific neuronal pattern is memorized, becoming the brain's concept of the visual aspect of the thumb. After verifying multiple deductions concerning the luminous characteristics of the body surface in this manner, brains must form general principles concerning visual signals: specific neuronal patterns represent linearity, others curves and so on in compulsive biocomputer detail. Having actively collected these principles, brains no longer need to verify all visual data by palpation. The shape of objects can be plotted with vision alone. For people hoping to understand consciousness, the crucial importance of the preceding is that patterns of neuronal variation in the visual cortex corresponding to luminous aspects of the body surface and later generalized for the purpose of visual monitoring, are meaningful for individual brains by reference to that brains' tactile symbols of the body surface, curves, lines etc. They are significant idiosyncratically only. That is why research involving the visual system can never explain what visual sensation is, let alone sensation pure and simple. Also, the neuronal symbolism for the visual aspects of body parts must be stored elsewhere than in the visual cortex, as must be neuronal symbolism for luminous patterns signifying lines, curves, volumes, cubes, cylinders etc. In brief, neuronal variations in the visual cortex become meaningful only after animal brains teach themselves tactile "sensation," the deduction of the meaning of said variations is downstream of the primary visual cortex, and all meaningful neuronal patterns are idiosyncratic to the brain the researcher is studying and ipso facto undecipherable by researchers. Monkeys' visual categorization of objects (as well as all animals') cannot be contained in the primary visual cortex. They are specific *concepts*, symbolic, and stored elsewhere in the neocortex. When the neocortex processes signals concerning previously categorized objects, recognition requires passage of bioelectric potentials along synaptic association tracts linking deductions downstream of the primary visual cortex with a data bank of categorized objects. Therefore, if there are neuronal variations in the prefrontal and inferior temporal cortices of brains of monkeys looking at dogs – as well as in the striate cortex – it is probable that the non-striate variations are not visual *sensations* nor visual *categories*. The temporal cortex variations might concern acoustic characteristics of dogs (barking) since the temporal operculi are the cortical foci of the "sensation" of sound (ergo synaptic visuo-auditory association about dogs). The prefrontal cortex variations might represent the symbolic concept "dog" pure and simple, synaptically linked to the contemporary visual deduction, "dog." Or, the prefrontal cortical variations might be neocortical control of eye movements (in human brains there are anterior frontal lobe centers controlling eye movements linked to the brainstem by the superior longitudinal fasciculus) and be distinct from visual "sensation," directing the search for visual targets.

In conclusion, evolution and embryology predetermine the order of acquisition of the individual "senses." In all cases, animals must acquire tactile sensation first, if they are to stand any chance of making sense out of variations in the primary long-distance sensory cortices (of elaborating long-distance sensory modalities). All long-distance sensory modalities first acquire meaning by reference to what brains have plotted as the corporal surface by logical processing involving the somesthetic-brain-muscle-brain feedback loop, the only "direct" sensory feedback loop available to the neocortex. After sufficient trials and data-averaging, brains form general symbolic concepts within each sensory modality allowing identification of distant objects using long-range "senses" only. But the first correlations of variations in the cortices of long-range senses with shapes of objects were those established when somesthetic and long-range cortical sensory variations concerned a same feature of the corporal envelope (knowing the linear and curved contours of the thumb by tactile exploration defines which patterns of visual cortex neuronal variations will be interpreted by brains as triggered by light reflected from linear and curved surfaces etc.) If the English word "hand" printed in letters of the Roman alphabet were a sensation (and therefore consisted of a precise neuronal pattern), then researchers seeking to understand consciousness and observing the neuronal pattern symbolizing "hand" written in Roman letters, would need to know that there exists a Roman alphabet, and would benefit from fluency in it. If they know only the Hebrew or Greek alphabets they could stare at the symbol for Roman-alphabet "hand" and never be the wiser – even more so if they were unaware that they were looking for symbols for a specific alphabet and were ignorant in *all* alphabets. People who try to understand sentience by restricting themselves to "research" on vision are like non-linguists (laymen) trying to "read" inscriptions in an unknown language of some newly-unearthed ruins of an unknown people while not aware that the inscriptions could fall into one of the multiple categories: ideograms, pictograms, cuneiform, hieroglyphic, or one of an infinity of possible alphabets. The letters for alphabets often stand for sounds in an original language. For example, "beth" in the Hebrew alphabet reproduces the sound for

Western Semitic "house" (bayit in Hebrew, bet in Aramaic and presumably something similar in the original Phoenician language). The Greek alphabet derives from the Phoenician and the Roman from the Greek. I don't know the Greek for "house" but suspect it is not the sound "beta," and the Latin "casa" certainly isn't the sound "bee" in Italian, French, or English – or Latin! In fact, vision is the only true long-range modality – the one most necessary to reference with tact. Snakes don't have ears but can detect sounds by vibrations against their skins. This is the macro analog of non-body matter contacting protozoan cell membranes. The same applies for long-range body-heat detection by snakes, echolocation by bats and dolphins and detection of bioelectricity by hammerhead sharks etc. So research alone – sans pondering the significance of data – and particularly research on the visual system cannot explain either visual sensation or sensation in general. For brains, the meaning of cortical neuronal variations is at first referential to the "somesthetic" data bank. Here is how:

There is ambient light. Eyelids are open (something the brain registers as: There is non-contact of eyelids). There are neuronal variations in the visual cortex which as yet are meaningless to the neocortex. Eyelids close. Brain registers: contact of lids. And, visual cortex neuronal variations cease. After multiple recurrences of these phenomena, the brain deduces that visual neuronal cortex variations (or: variation phenomena "x," since it is unaware of neurons and brain anatomy and doesn't yet have a label for phenomenon "x") are non-contact signals. Now, eyes are oriented in the sector of space that contains the thumb (we know the position of our thumb even with eyes shut). There is light and non-contact of eyelids. Visual cortex neuronal variations commence. Some concern the thumb. Eyes and thumb are ordered to move together through space. Some visual cortex variations (those concerning the thumb) remain relatively unchanged throughout all displacements. Eyelids are made to open and close randomly. Whenever they close, all visual cortical variations, including those about the thumb, disappear. Data-averaging and analysis of multiple, repeated, simultaneous somesthetic, kinesthetic, proprioceptive and visual (cortical) variations conclude that one kind of variation (later experienced as "vision") occurs only when palpebral muscles are relaxed and eyelids not in contact. Therefore, these variations happen only when there is non-contact of lids. Let tact or somesthesia, previously discovered to mean "contact," be symbolized by "C." Then those variations occurring only when eyelids are open are "non-C" ($\sim$ C). And if "touch" materially equals "contact" (terms of formal logic – $T \equiv C$) the second category of as–yet meaningless variations (X) corresponds materially to non-contact or: $X \equiv \sim C$. Multiple trials with thumb held before eyes establish which portions of the total "X" variation pattern pertain to the thumb. They become meaningful by reference to the somesthetic concept of the thumb but once they are meaningful, they may be applied to plot non-thumb visual variations concerning non-body macroscopic items. But data-averaging also establishes that when there is a non-contact of eyelids visual (cortical) variations sometimes take place and sometimes not (always binary logic!). Merely opening eyelids is therefore insufficient, in and of itself, to cause variations in the visual cortex. There must, therefore exist a variable (call it "L" for light) whose present is required in addition to non-contact of eyelids, if there are to be visual-cortical variations. "L" (light) becomes real by circular reasoning: brains must conclude that when lids are open and visual-cortex variations occur, light is present while absence of visual-cortical variations means it is absent. The physical variable necessary to experience visual-cortical variations is "light" or "L," and the "sensation" it provides is "vision." From this point the logic cascade (proceeding in symbolic binary mode) must continue as follows:

1. $V \neq S$ (Vision is not somesthesia, or tact)
2. $V \neq K$ (Vision is not kinesthesia, or: it is not muscle activity)
3. $\Delta V = f\,O\,x$
4. $Ox = f\,\Delta\,EOM$
3. Variations in the visual cortex are a function of the orientation of devices x (the ocular globes).
4. The orientation of devices (x) – the eyeballs – is a function of variations of the extraocular muscles.

Determining the functional significance of cortical olfactory, gustatory and auditory variations is an application of the same logical binary cascade for each modality: when a same item simultaneously causes cortical somesthetic, visual, auditory, gustatory and olfactory variations, some neuronal patterns of each modality must concern an aspect of the item. With somesthetic and visual neocortical variations both understood, repeated reproductions of variations concerning the item in each sensory modality remaining will allow exclusion of non-item variations (which don't recur consistently throughout the repeated trials) as non-item caused. The neuronal variation pattern reproduced most often (and more so if always) is the auditory, olfactory or gustatory symbol for the item. Schematically, visual variations symbolizing an item "x" are the non-contact, non-auditory, non-gustatory and non-olfactory symbolic variations concerning "x" when "x" triggers all peripheral detectors simultaneously:

$V\,x = ({\sim}\,C, {\sim}\,A, {\sim}\,G, {\sim}\,O)x$ (~ is the symbol in formal logic for "non"). The brain's symbolic definition of all other non-contact, non-vision sensations is a general one in which the sensory modality is left of the equation and all others are enclosed in the parentheses on the right. If all the preceding is valid, then symbolic neocortical processing is not only one of binary logic (x or non-x) but also of symbolic neuronal integral calculus.

The relative enhancement of security neurons derive from the multicellular stratagem comes at the cost of relative facility in obtaining food at the microscopic level. The cell membrane of protozoa can assimilate food, but since the envelope of the multicellular collective is relatively impenetrable to microscopic assault (the reason *for* multicellularity), openings must be introduced in the envelope and means developed to introduce food through the openings. Solutions are either a permanent or voluntary opening in skin. The location and orientation of these apertures is vital to know. It must be localized in a first (discovery) phase and monitored thereafter when mealtimes come. If the location at the moment is established it can be propelled at food in any of several ways involving commands to muscles, or food can be brought to it by tentacles or limbs. A derivative tactic is the active search for food by displacement of the entire multicellular collective. This creates the need for means of locomotion. Now, it is one thing to lead relatively stationary lives (like barnacles and sea anemones) attached either to rocks or to mobile animals (e.g. whales), passively filtering water with tentacles and transporting the catch to the mouth. Jellyfish, which are animal colonies, practice a variant of this, flowing in currents to secure food encountered by chance. It is quite another mathematical and bioengineering challenge to actively pursue food. This requires means of displacement manipulated as such by the neocortex, under cortical control. Also mandatory is appreciation of the milieu in which displacements occur. Appreciating milieus and controlling displacements in them necessitate neuronal deductions effected according to logical/mathematical principles. This is the specialization of the neocortex. But the first-formed and functioning nervous *system* (i.e. the first integrated neuronal circuit system of and in multicellular animals) is an unconscious ("vegetative") one. Its mission is monitoring the chemical status within the body and maintaining it between optimal ranges. Its peripheral and central components work together in a feedback servo-mechanism fashion. By ensuring optimal chemical conditions for the body's organs and tissues while the immune system staves off microscopic threats, this system provides optimal support of cerebral neurons. The system's central component is the chemical, or autonomic brain. In humans it maintains a blood pH of 7.35 to 7.45, optimal arterial/venous 02 and C02 concentrations, blood sugar between 80 and 126 mg %, etc. To achieve homeostasis the vegetative system is arranged so that some parts do assays (of sugar, blood pH, p02 and pC02, electrolyte concentrations etc) while others transmit commands correcting aberrations. These commands from the central component to effector components are (a) chemical: hormones are released into the circulation on command, modifying organ activities and consequently the chemical milieu in relatively long times, and (b): bioelectric potentials relayed along sympathetic or parasympathetic nerves to specific organs, modifying their activities instantly and thus, too, the chemical milieu. Both the hormonal and electrically induced changes affect organs *in* the body – those with mechanical missions (heart and respiratory muscles for example) and those with chemical ones (thyroid, kidneys, pancreas...). These organs are firmly anchored in the coelome by membranes and ligaments. It is not necessary to monitor their locations. In early life before age takes its toll, we are unaware of these organs. If we survive long enough to have heart attacks, liver damage, or spinal nerve root compressions, then the affected organs relay "damage!" (pain) signals to the brain along tracts shared with the left arm, right shoulder, and thigh-leg-and-foot (for the lumbosacral nerve roots) so that the brain, accustomed to damage signals from left arm, right shoulder, and legs mistakes the provenance of the new signals.

Target organs for hormones act entirely by chemical means – kidneys (hormone: ADH), thyroid (TSH), pancreas (IRF – insulin releasing factor), adrenals (ACTH) etc. But some internal organs regulating the chemical composition of the internal environment do so mechanically as well as chemically: lungs, heart, blood vessels. Their mechanical performance is modulated by cerebral electric potentials relayed in sympathetic and parasympathetic nerves. Thus, pulmonary regulation of pH, p02 and pCo2 is modified by cerebral commands via the phrenic and intercostal nerves to the diaphragm and intercostal muscles, adjusting rates and strength of contraction of these muscles. As a consequence lungs fill or empty of air more or less quickly and voluminously.

Central commands via specific autonomic nerves also alter the rate and force of cardiac contractions, and thus adjust systemic blood flow and pressure. Similar autonomic control of vascular constriction or dilatation is exerted via sympathetic nerves, while the vagus nerve transmits potentials adjusting gastrointestinal motility. Phylogenetically as well as ontogenetically (heart and blood vessels start working in embryos), autonomic (vegetative) electric transactions are a prelude or apprenticeship for neocortex-body electrical transactions with the body surface and non-body macroscopic world. If two-way electrical exchanges suffice as an exchange-medium between internal organs and vegetative brain, the system constitutes a model for exchanges between the body surface and the neocortex. It remains simply to discover the rules of exchange and adapt them to the supra-autonomic nervous system. These rules concern the values and functional significance of electrical exchanges and the symbolic neuronal logical processes that enable obligated users of this exchange system to discover said rules.

Brain cells are separated from the macro environment by tissues of species – in invertebrates, by soft tissues only or a combination of soft tissues and exoskeleton. In humans, by the meninges, inner and outer tables of the skull, galea and scalp. Data about macro phenomena is collected by peripheral tissues differentiated into finite organs detecting specific aspects of macro matter/energy. The principles of macroscopic biologic detection were itemized on pages 52, 53, 59, 73, 83-84, and 94-95. We must always bear in mind that neuronal circuits in brains never encounter nor receive, and cannot form literal versions of the contents of the macro world since light and sound are absent in brains. The matter/energy at neurons' disposal allows them to form synaptic links and cell-circuits and to vary in electric state but not to erect models of macroscopic phenomena. Rather, variations in electrical state are "exploited" to build a symbolic conceptual library of items deduced to exist in the universe after symbolic processing of second-hand data (data signaled by non-neuronal elements of the multicellular collective). Detection by biological systems is active and dynamic and requires operation of all system-elements: peripheral detectors, tracts to brains, relay of bioelectricity along the tracts when detectors are triggered, neuronal variations in the cortices receiving signals and processing of neocortical signal-induced variations by downstream cell circuits. If components are missing or the system does not work in the correct sequence or manner then the presence and/or operation of elements in isolation is cognitively useless. A pool of water may reflect light, but absent relay of some signal to a processing unit (tracts which relay molecules, bioelectricity, sound etc and thus induce electrical or mechanical variations monitored and processed downstream of the reception area *when the pool reflects light*), the pool is not a detecting device. The same is true of echo chambers so long as they only bounce sound waves. Or, if the surfaces of two rocks come in contact but this is not signaled, the contact is not the sensation "tact." What makes something a detector is not its power of resolution, but the transmission of some form of signal allowing a receiving unit to deduce the device was triggered. Since all detectors of macro phenomena send the *same* kind of signal (a bioelectric potential), brains must discover via symbolic deductive logic what triggers each organ of detection. We have enumerated and given the sequence of the deductive process. Now, detection and deductions by nervous systems is not done for art's sake, but to promote survival. Survival cannot be assured if detections and analysis are intermittent and random. They must be continuous. Therefore, nervous systems are organized and integrated for scanning (monitoring). Survival is better served by continuous monitoring regardless of poor resolution, than by detection in exquisite detail performed randomly and in spurts. Photographs reveal greater or lesser detail depending on grain, but document only aspects of nature frozen in time and usually irrelevant to circumstances at the times they are viewed. Constant visual scanning by healthy systems yields data of more existential import than the most detailed photograph. As for the vocabulary of cognitive symbolism:

When thumb and lips juxtapose, we say, "I touched my lip with my thumb." If voluntary, the event was preceded by formulation and execution of *intent* to appose the two. The word "touch" is, then, a verb: past tense of "to touch." Hoary tradition and lack of knowledge of neurobiology prior to the 1890's allowed a semantic and conceptual corruption whereby the verb is also used as a noun: "touch" as an autonomous *thing* or *item*, designated an order and form of sentience: consciousness of the fact of touching, but not yet perception (the next order of sentience). Other noun corruptions of verbs are "sight," "hearing," "smell" and "taste." When it is a matter of sensory modalities not present in humans, there are no such linguistic perversions – what are the noun-forms of the "sensations" of echolocation, thermal detection, bioelectric detection? Snakes may "see" rodents in the verb sense of "see," so we say they have "sight," using "sight" as a noun. We know they can also detect rodents' body heat, but we don't say they have "heat," where "heat" is used as a noun. We recognize that bats and dolphins can "see," but we don't refer to their echolocation activities as "radaring." In other words, actions such as seeing or hearing are labeled "sensations," each corresponding to a modality of the general category "feeling" where "feeling" is used as a noun. But brains don't "feel" thumbs and lips "touching" and thumbs and lips decidedly have no "feelings." The reality is that integrated neuronal-circuit processings culminated in logical *deductions* that there were triggerings at points of a periphery neurons can never personally "feel," "see," "touch," etc of organs primed for activation by juxtaposed surfaces; the triggered organs are situated on the surface of what brains previously plotted to be "their" thumb and lips: the spatial location of these body parts is monitored by kinesthetic/proprioceptive "sensations" and they are apposed. Ergo: *they are triggering each other.* It has been shown intraoperatively that the brain itself does not "feel." Unless incisions, cauterizations, mechanical or electrical stimuli are made at specific, pin-point locations in the brain (identical in all brains), the brain ignores stimuli. When certain areas are stimulated, specific responses ensue. Stimulating specific parts of the motor strip causes variations of muscles in predictable parts of the body. Stimulating specific locations in the somesthetic strip produces hallucinations of "touch" in predictable body sites. Striate cortex stimulation causes unformed visual hallucinations while stimulating parts of the thalamus causes hallucinations of pain localized to controlateral body segments. Hallucinations are therefore neuronal variations in specific cerebral loci occurring in the absence of normal instigations of said variations. The normal instigators are potentials arriving from peripheral organs which were actually triggered by contact, light, sound, or molecular stimuli (nasal mucosa and taste buds). "Sensations" that skin is being contacted or light or sound being registered at the periphery are occurring *without* corresponding peripheral events. Brains producing hallucinations are not monitoring ("sensing") actual events happening at the periphery but *mimicking* neuronal deductions concerning actual peripheral phenomena. Intraoperative or pathologic stimulation of cerebral neurons in particular regions produce *illusions* of actual variations of the organs normally stimulating the brain area which is being *abnormally* active. The body and its parts have no "feelings." Blocking signals following actual stimulation of sense organs with local anesthetics or sometimes simply by applying tourniquets downstream of the stimulated organ allows brains to remain alert, yet be unaware of the dental drilling or sutures being placed in skin. We feel no "pain" nor "touch." "Feelings" or "sensations" are therefore only more-or-less valid neuronal deductions which normally result from cerebral neuronal circuits' processing of signals from sense organs which were actually triggered. Sans actual triggering of detectors, relay and reception of signals and actual processing of signal-induced sensory cortex variations, these deductions could not have formed a first time. Deductions that skin is contacting matter, surfaces reflect light and sound and so on are not "feelings" – a deduction is a deduction is a deduction. Since they are not literal copies of extracerebral items – intracranial replicas in light, sound, and matter of macroscopic items outside brains and even outside bodies – they are symbolic deductions, made of synaptically linked neurons, *that* specific macroscopic phenomena are triggering specific peripheral detectors. Once brains actively discover and define for themselves every sensory modality they own, and as occurrences of each newly understood sensation become familiar through repetition, each primary deduction (i.e. each "sensation," the hierarchical preceder of perceptions) acquires an individual "personality." Sensations qua personalities are unique and therefore recognizable. When things acquire recognition in their own right through frequent encounters, it is no longer necessary to go through the ascending logic cascade each time another macro phenomenon is signaled via that sensation and deduce ad infinitum that it is none of the other sensations. As an "I"-input, it is now *part* of "I." That fact of becoming familiar increases the speed with which brains can monitor the world. The "personalities" are symbolic abbreviations for the sensations. It is these "personalities" that we experience as "feelings" (tact, sight and our other sensations) yet they are merely symbolic abbreviations for symbolic deductions, rendering scanning more efficient by shaving nanoseconds off time which would otherwise be consumed processing received signals. Empirical support for this thesis (as well as for the speed with which neocortical circuits process data, a subject treated at some length earlier in this manuscript) is contained in an article in "Neurology Reviews" which appeared in March, 2001.[5]

"Neurons in the ventral prefrontal cortex 'see' danger and start firing off warning signals long before there is any conscious awareness of fear, according to research reported by Hiroto Kawasaki, Ph.D., and colleagues in the January issue of Nature Neuroscience. The University of Iowa research team found that neurons in the ventromedial frontal cortex perform a very rapid, coarse sorting of stimulus emotional content within 120 to 160-ms of stimulus sighting and quickly respond to stimuli related to fear, threat, or danger. According to co-author Ralph Adolphs... 'An aversive stimulus triggered a short-latency, transient inhibition, which was followed by prolonged excitation. We think these neurons categorize stimuli to which the organism needs to mount a rapid response... The evolutionary argument would be that these are situations in which we need to move promptly out of harm's way, even before we are consciously aware of being afraid.'"

---

5. "Prefrontal Cortex Neurons Give Early Warning Of Danger," March, 2001, p.p. 10-11

Now, the words, "consciously aware" mean the same thing. One is either aware (conscious) of something, or not. One cannot be conscious (i.e. aware) of things before becoming aware (conscious) of them. The phrases "consciously unaware" or "aware unconsciously" are oxymoronic and nonsensical. In the study, subjects were shown "aversive stimuli" such as pictures of mutilated bodies. Recording electrodes implanted in their brain documented, 120 to 160-ms after exposure, the frontal lobe activity preceding the emotional response. That frontal neuronal variation could *not* be fear the subjects were as yet unconscious of having (an oxymoron). It has to be the *perception* (a neuronal deduction one step after sensations in the ascending logic cascade) that visual data concern mutilated bodies. The emotional response is *contingent* on perception, which is the recognition of the significance of the sensory data (what the data means). The merit of this research is that it proves that intracortical neuronal processing is very fast. 120 to 160-ms after exposure to visual stimuli, neuronal processing has identified the visual data as mutilated bodies. The visual cortex neuronal variations did not have to be distinguished from variations occurring simultaneously in the somesthetic, auditory and other "sensory" cortices because visual variations are recognizable as such by "I" and the time needed to pass from "sensation" to perception was accordingly shortened. This obtains because after innumerable "by the book," step-by-symbolic step processing of visual signals, cortical neuronal visual variations are invested with personality for "I" and biologic computer operations can be abbreviated.

Machines are material expressions of a logic, or a set of principles. That logic is the active, specific and explicit modification of matter/energy. Qualitatively, quantitatively or in combination, forms of matter and energy (or combinations of both) are modified into different forms. Machines are matter/energy modifiers. Its success or failure validates or invalidates the principles and logic governing a particular machine. If the components and inputs are known and the products approximately known, it is possible to deduce how the components are organized and interact to produce the product. Correct deductions concerning the manufacturing process clarify the nature of the product. Imagine a contemporary hunter-gatherer newly exposed to automobiles but incapable of distinguishing trucks from sedans or Toyotas from Fords. An automobile factory opens nearby. He is barred entry, but can observe in exquisite detail the entry of raw materials to the factory and the exit, later, of sedans, RUVs and pickup trucks, all Fords. He might surmise that metallic ores are converted to metal sheets in foundries and then various machines inside the building. He might surmise that a liquid is transformed chemically and mechanically into rubber tires, etc. And, he might learn the differences between sedans, pickups and RUVs. By observing finished vehicles exiting the Ford plant he might, if encountering them, distinguish Toyota vehicles from their Ford analogs.

The machines which produce consciousness are nervous systems. If members of a species never develop a sensory modality belonging in their species, it must be because their nervous systems have defects or didn't function post-nataly before the deadline for forming that modality ("Use it or lose it" is advice for *retaining* capacities or assets in old age, but is just as true as concerns post-natal cognitive development). People who become blind or deaf after living part of their lives with sight and hearing can't monitor the *contemporary* world with visual/auditory systems, but have concepts of light and sound and audiovisual data banks. Their occipital and temporal lobe neuronal circuits defining light and sound were formed and had functioned before their disabilities were incurred. Conversely, people and other animals born with non-functioning audiovisual *systems* (whether the flaw lie in the organ of detection, its links to the neocortex, the neocortex itself or any combination of these) never form audiovisual concepts or data banks. More: if the defects are peripheral and correctable (cataracts; ear infections) they may acquire the sensory modality if the condition is diagnosed and corrected in time, but not if correction is done after the deadline for forming that modality – or, in the latter case, limited but not full audiovisual sentience might develop.

If corrections must be made before a deadline age while corrections performed after it provide people with technically adequate eyes and ears yet they remain blind and deaf, then their failure to acquire sentience must be because of either non-formation or non-functioning of neocortical neuronal circuits.

The corollary of this is that neocortical cell-circuits must have formed as well as functioned for sensory modalities to form, and there is a time limit for forming and using circuits. Natural selection and embryology cause the neocortex to enter the post-incubation world with neurons disposed in vertical and horizontal layers. Cell-circuits are made up of neurons linked by synapses vertically, horizontally or both. There is a post-natal time window for forming these synapses. After it has passed, these synapses will not form. Why must synapses form by a deadline age? Because synapses are what makes circuits possible. If synapses haven't formed by the critical age they will not, and circuits will not have formed – and neuronal circuits are the machines producing sentience. Now we are born with all the gray matter (neurons) we will have in our lives. Yet the human brain weighs about 350 grams at birth but increases to its lifetime maximum of about 1300 grams around two years of age. The increased weight and volume are due entirely to white-matter formation. White matter (glial cells) plays a structural support and immunologic role in brains. It also has what is theorized as a "sink action:" variations in neuronal electrical state are accomplished by exchanges of sodium and potassium between cells and their external milieu, and releases of chemical mediators at synaptic clefts. It is speculated that glia (white matter) dispose of excess mediators and electrolytes. An article in the journal "science" describes a fourth role played by glia – a role which (if true) accounts for the need to form circuits by a certain age: [6].

"... few synapses form in the absence of glial cells and the few synapses that do form are functionally immature. Astrocytes increase the number of mature, functional synapses on central nervous system (CNS) neurons by sevenfold and are required for synaptic maintenance in vitro... most synapses are generated concurrently with the development of glia in vivo. These data demonstrate a previously unknown function for glia in inducing and stabilizing CNS synapses..."

The four-fold increase in brain weight after birth is due entirely to glial increase. On page 569 of that issue of "Science" it is stated that glia constitute 90% of cells in the brain. This means that roughly 75% of glia appear post-birth. The gray/white appearance of infant brains on MRI (Magnetic Resonance Imaging) approaches that of adult brains toward roughly two years of age. The bulk of glial formation must therefore be accomplished around that age. It is documented that non-correction of congenital end-organ disease (e.g. strabismus; cataracts) prior to 2, 3, or 4 years of age always entails non-acquisition of part or all of a sensory modality (vision in the case of cataracts; depth-perception in the case of strabismus). The completion of myelination must, accordingly, preclude significant new circuit formation and if Ullian, Sapperstein et al are correct the reason is that initial and fundamental synapse and circuit formation occur in tandem with glial formation. Unlike neurons, glia are replaceable but the maximal num-

---

6. "Control of Synapse Number by Glia," E.M. Ullian, S.K. Sapperstein et al, Science, Vol. 291 No. 5504, 26 Jan., 2001, p.p. 657-659

ber is fixed at age two or thereabouts. Ergo, neocortical synapses and circuits fundamental for sensation are established around age two and cannot form after. If synaptic formation is proportional to glial volume and is not inhibited at a critical glial volume, the mind boggles at the intellectual ramifications of prolonging the period of glial formation. In any case, if circuits are considered machines for processing bioelectricty, we can hypothesize symbolic circuits by combining excitatory and inhibitory neurons. The following circuit models function according to Boolean logic. They are not submitted as the *only* possible processing mechanism, but the author is unable to imagine other symbolic mechanisms. An article in "Science" suggests that single neurons in an owl's inferior colliculus act "like an 'and' gate." (In said piece, ILD is an abbreviation for interaural level difference while ITD means interaural time difference):[7]

"Two properties illustrate what it means for a neuron to multiply. First, when very faint ITD and ILD signals correspond to the same region of space (giving mutually affirming indications that a mouse is underneath a log off to the right, say) neurons in the inferior colliculus fire robustly. If the two subthreshold signals were added, in contrast, their combined stimulation wouldn't rile up the space-specific neurons enough to fire. Second, the lack of either an ITD or an ILD signal can veto a space-specific neuron's firing. In multiplication, 2x0 = 0; in a barn owl's

7. Location Neurons Do Advances Math, Science, 13 April 2001, Vol. 292 No. 5515 p. 185

inferior colliculus, a strong ITD signal x no ILD signal = no response. As Peña explains, the neuron acts like an "and" gate, requiring both signals, rather than an "or" gate, which could respond to just one." Now, this is an "and" gate in a very limited sense: the neuron responds to either temporal or spatial summation or possibly both. But to also have "or" and "not" gates, single neurons are not sufficient – only *circuits* combining excitatory and inhibitory cells fit the bill. Since light, sound, trees, comets, birds etc do not exist in heads yet we know they exist, our knowledge is a matter of symbolic concepts consisting of synapses uniting groups of neurons themselves resulting (i.e. designated meaningful) from symbolic operations of other, synaptically-linked neuronal circuits. The "machines" (symbolic-logical processing units of bioelectricity) might not perform *Boolean* logic but *must* consist of symbolic combinations of excitatory and inhibitory neurons. Conventionally, excitatory neurons are designated Golgi type I and inhibitory neurons Golgi type II cells. Appropriate synaptic combinations of the two can form circuits functioning as Boolean "and," "or" and "not" gates (I reiterate that neuronal logic might be other than Boolean and want only to show that synapses between Golgi I and II cells can constitute symbolic logical processors of bioelectricity; I haven't the time to invent other logic systems). It is possible to form any combination of gates and any number of circuits. Also, Golgi I and II cells may be combined to form memory bits and used to retrieve same. And, the two sorts of neurons suffice to transmit commands to muscles.

The exclusive currency of all transactions to, in and from the neocortex is the bioelectric potential. It is created through exchange of intracellular potassium with extracellular sodium, resulting in potentials in the mini-to-microvolt range. Received potentials are converted to cognition by processing through logic circuits while transmitting potentials are commands to previously identified striated muscles. Received and transmitted potentials are *rendered* existentially meaningful by active, symbolic neocortical circuit operations.

The first incoming "sensory" potentials must engage IS-WAS immediate memory circuits. This enables downstream circuits to deduce that there has been variation in the (electrical) state of neocortical receptor neurons (in fact, their only possible deduction is that something varied – they can never know that *neurons* are what varies). Processing by yet further-downstream circuits deduces particular "sensations" while in some species even further processing yields perceptions. Superior circuits monitoring logical operations occurring simultaneously when more than one sensory modality is triggered by non-body phenomena sort out separate sensory modalities. Perceptions (in normal humans) are products of logical circuit-operations one order of magnitude less than ideas (which are logically more complex than perceptions which are more complex than sensations). Given sufficient neurons and sufficient, additional primary circuit formation it is hard to imagine an end-point to what might be intellectually possible. In fact, end points of a general order *are* reached within animal species and characterize the species as a whole (whales are more intelligent than swine which are more intelligent than bovines etc) although these end-points appear quite disparate between members of a same species (individuals differ in ability to "sense," perceive and reason).

Functional Significance of Circuits

One way of categorizing cells is by their action: muscle cells elongate or shorten, endocrine cells synthesize and secrete hormones and neurons receive, generate and transmit bioelectric potentials. If neocortical receptor neurons and some of their downstream circuits vary on receiving potentials from the body surface, these variations are directly related to the triggered organ at the surface. If the sequential peripheral variations of polysynaptic reflexes are echoed by sequential variations of neocortical neurons and circuits linked to each peripheral element, then the neocortical variations are directly proportional to the polysynaptic ones. If a "superior" circuit-system deduces that one set of variations invariably precedes another set (or sub-set), a fourth circuit system may deduce that the first variation induces the second. If other circuits could voluntarily command muscle contractions, yet others may deduce that something (muscle activity) may be caused by "I" or by "non-I."

The initial discovery (of the envelope, i.e. skin of the body) and of the non-body macro universe results from processing of electrical transactions between three cell types: cells of cutaneous mechanoreceptors, striated muscle cells, and neurons. Retinal rods and cones (light detectors), cochlear "hair" cells (sound detectors), nasal and lingual cells detecting molecules are not elements of reflex loops which include neocortical neurons. Consequently they cannot serve to make deductions about time/space, the existence of the corporal envelope or the non-body universe (which is why research confined to macroscopic non-contact senses cannot explain how sentience arises nor what sentience is). But given segmental reflex arcs between cutaneous mechanoreceptors, muscles having sensory relays to the neocortex and the neocortical ability to activate the same muscles contracting reflexly to triggering of mechanoreceptors in skin, neocortical cell-circuits can deduce the following:

1. That "I" cause something to vary.
2. That "I" can simultaneously cause variations of several different somethings.
3. That responses to my simultaneous activations of specific different somethings arrive in immutable and fixed sequential orders despite the simultaneous activations, and the sequence never varies between specific somethings (muscles).
4. These fixed, sequential latencies constitute "I's" definition of TIME.
5. If times of response are variable (muscles are variably distant from "I") but constant for specific variables (specific muscles) then there is something called SPACE.
6. The somethings "I" cause to vary are spatially removed from "I" *because* they are removed in time.

7. When the somethings vary but I did not command variation, their variations must be caused by something(s) which is/are "non-I."

The important thing to realize is that the preceding are *deductions* by neuronal *circuits*. Circuits can't "sense" but can calculate. Individual neurons can neither "sense" *nor* calculate (contrary to the hypothesis of "and" or "multiplication" neurons). Neocortical cell-circuits are symbolic machines which process a single raw material: the bioelectric potential.

We have proposed some of the logical/symbolic processing neuronal circuits *must* make if brains are to acquire competence in appreciating the macro environment and in maneuvering the body in that environment. The precise, arbitrary sequence of steps was reasoned out in function of the material resources, physical connections, and physiology which mandate which steps, and in what order, are possible.

In the current state of technology we either cannot observe or have not systematically and compulsively traced the totality of synapses a neuron establishes with other neurons. At least one author puts the number at around one thousand:

"The brain has about a hundred billion neurons, each connected to about a thousand other cells; simply producing any sort of a wiring diagram is a monumental project." [8]

However, once it is accepted that some synapses have got to combine excitatory and inhibitory neu-

8. David C. Noelle, op. cit.

rons into circuits which function symbolically and make binary logical deductions (Boolean or not) the *experimental* project should be simplified – it is all a question of knowing what to look for. Researchers could begin by looking at primary receptor cortices for 4-neuron circuits representing symbolic IS-WAS (immediate memory) "wiring diagrams." I have argued that "sensations," command of striated muscles and Mind are *products* of symbolic logical operations at the histologic (neuronal) level, for neocortical data are received, processed and retained in the form of *variations* of neuronal electrical states. The data supporting the ascending logic cascade are, in the first instance, *chronologic*, the temporal relations between neuronal variations in cerebral space being the only phenomena measurable (i.e. comparable) for downstream circuits. The symbolic mechanism processing data consisting of neocortical neuronal variations has *got* to be a neuronal collective enterprise (ergo cell-circuits) because individual neurons cannot count, compare nor make deductions. Circuits are symbolically meaningful structural/dynamic neuronal *fusions* because there is nothing other than neurons in the neocortex permitting data-processing. The analytical method consisted of reasoning out what theorems/propositions can and must be discovered by neocortical circuits – given available histologic, neuroanatomic and physiologic data – so that, after additional circuits validate said theorems/propositions, "I" deduces that it is enclosed in a multicellular/tissular organism which is a material item of a macroscopic universe. Like all material systems, neocortical cell circuits must *express* symbolic-logical theorems in a materially symbolic manner.

I have argued that the neocortex is a biologic computer mediating inputs from peripheral "sense" organs with output in the form of commands to striated muscles, all in the form of bioelectric potentials. Its goal is ensuring neuronal survival in the macro universe by optimizing the survivability of the multicellular being containing neurons. It must discover the existence of "I," the body surface, and the non-body (or non-I) world. It must classify the non-body items it encounters as beneficial, hazardous or lethal, and indifferent. It is thus different from man-made computers by virtue of its raison d'être (promoting survival), the fact of having to program itself, and of having to address only three survival imperatives. Of course, since the numbers of benevolent, dangerous and indifferent environmental items are practically infinite, the survival goal is an expression of ultimate "ambition." The inner "wiring" of this protoplasmic computer must necessarily include symbolic logic elements (in the form of neuronal circuits) never dreamed of by human designers of inorganic computers. But since neuronal circuits process bioelectricity symbolically, there has to be *some* analogy with the symbolism and mechanics of man-made computers. To justify my hypotheses concerning neuronal circuit logic and symbolism I therefore recall some fundamentals of computer theory:

There are three kinds of computer: analog, digital and hybrid. The first measures, the second counts specifically or discretely, and the third is a combination of both. Analog computers represent the values of variables or numbers by physical quantities such as angular position or voltages. Digital computers count by responding, or not responding, to signals (that exist, or do not exist). Thus, the components of a digital computer (e.g. transistors or circuits) either conduct, or do not conduct; electric currents are pulsed, or not pulsed; areas of plastic tape are magnetized, or not magnetized. Any material, consistent event and non-event, or action and counteraction, can be *assigned* the symbolic values; one and zero. Arithmetically, the numbers one and zero suffice to perform any desired calculation, provided the calculation be effected according to a suitable arithmetic method. One such method is the binary system, in which any number can be represented by a combination of ones and zeros. Finally, the truth of falseness of any proposition can be established by submitting propositions to a method of algebraic and logical analysis developed by the mathematician George Boole in the 19th century, and expanded by another Englishman, Alan Turing, in the 1930's. In this method, all "trues" and "falses" can be processed by three logical functions, called AND, OR and NOT. These functions can be symbolized by 1's and 0's. Thus, it is materially possible to perform *both* logic *and* arithmetic with a material system wherein consistent actions and counteractions symbolize 1's and 0's.

The gist of the preceding paragraph is summarized by four tables which I copied in 1978. Unfortunately, the sources were misplaced so I cannot credit the author(s).

Table 1: Binary Numbers Represented By Actions and Counteractions

0	1
Zero voltage	Positive voltage
No current	Current
Negative pulse	Positive pulse
Low voltage	High Voltage
Zero voltage	Negative Voltage
No pulse	Pulse

Table 2: Basic Rules

Symbol	Logic	Relay or Contact	Meaning	Circuit
1	True	Closed	Statement is true, the circuit is closed.	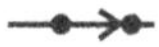
0	False	Open	Statement is false, the circuit is open.	
-	Series	A and B	A is in series with B.	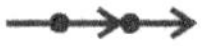
+	Parallel	A or B	A is in parallel with B.	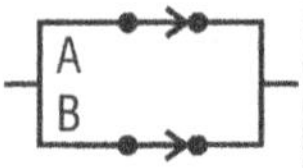
A	Not A		Opposite of A (if A = 0, A = 1 if A = 1, A = 0)	

Table 3: Series Circuits

Logic	Meaning	Circuit
0.0 = 0	An open in series with an open is open.	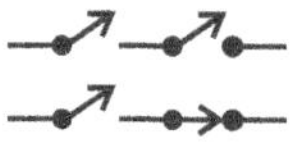
0.1 = 0	An open in series with a closed is open.	
1.1 = 1	A closed in series with a closed is closed.	
A.A = 0	A switch in series with its negation is open.	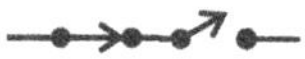

Table 4: Parallel Circuits

Logic	Meaning	Circuit
0 + 0 = 0	An open in parallel with an open is open.	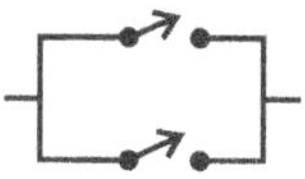
0 + 1 = 0	An open in parallel with a closed is closed.	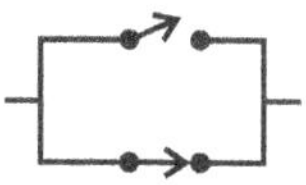
1 + 1 = 1	A closed in parallel with a closed is closed.	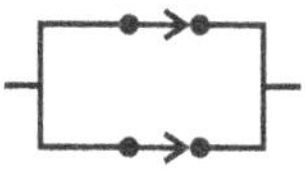
A + A = 1	A switch in parallel with its negation is closed.	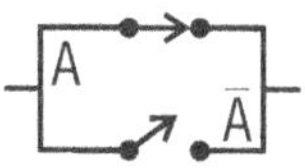

If we accept that the neocortex is a biological computer, then its neuronal component must be organized in some way which is functionally analogous to one or several of the circuits, relays and contacts detailed in the above tables. With said circuits and their only input (bioelectric potentials) data can be processed using combinations of And, Or and Not logic gates. Calculations can be performed by binary arithmetic or some other system consistent with the symbolic circuit reality.

Golgi I (excitatory neurons) activate neurons they synapse with while Golgi II (inhibitory) neurons deactivate neurons they synapse with. I propose that given adequate numbers of the two kinds of neurons, all requisite circuits may form, all existentially vital logical/arithmetic processing be conducted, and all the orders of sentience be elaborated. There is no question that the number of neurons in the neocortex is more than adequate. It remains simply to show some organization (wiring) possibilities. For starters, we must think of how Golgi I and II neurons might be combined to form switches causing potentials to enter either one or another circuit, and also causing either flow or non-flow of bioelectric currents. This was shown earlier in previous manuscripts (neuronal single and double switches, see Appendix on page 167). Second, we must imagine how the two sorts of neurons might combine to produce currents that either pulsate, or do not pulsate (and therefore serve to count by binary I's and O's). here is one possibility:

The Pulsating Circuit

When a given flexor muscle (e.g. the biceps brachii) contracts, its extensor antagonist (here, the triceps brachii) relaxes, and vice-versa. Inactive muscles generate bioelectric potentials at frequencies designated “baseline.” This frequency increases with contraction of muscles and decreases with lengthening (relaxation). All such variations are relayed to the sensorimotor (muscle-sensory) cortex causing receptor neurons in said cortex to vary. Variations of agonist/antagonist muscle couples are inversely proportional. The inverse proportionality can be exploited by combining Golgi I and II neurons in such fashion as to form a pulsating circuit. The circuit has a terminal which is always either open or closed. Whenever it is open, current cannot flow downstream while when it is closed there is flow. It is *always* open when flexors contract and *always* closed when extensors relax (or the reverse. Which case applies might be predetermined by evolution and embryology; or, the determination could be idiosyncratic, one case obtaining in some members of a species and the other in the remainder). An open terminal has the neuronal and computer symbolic value binary zero while a closed terminal has the significance: binary 1. Accordingly, if terminals are open only when x flexor motor units vary, the sum equals x binary zeros. When y extensor motor units vary, the sum equals y binary 1’s. Arithmetic additions of x’s and y’s are made by neuronal half-adders and full-adders (half adders are the basic counting units [or circuits] of computers. All computer arithmetic is performed by suitable numbers of half and full-adders. How neurons might form half-adders will be shown shortly).

Since the fetal position is flexed, it seems reasonable to postulate that flexion is the binary zero state. The pulsating circuit we shall now hypothesize is therefore one where flexion is the binary zero state (Figure 8).

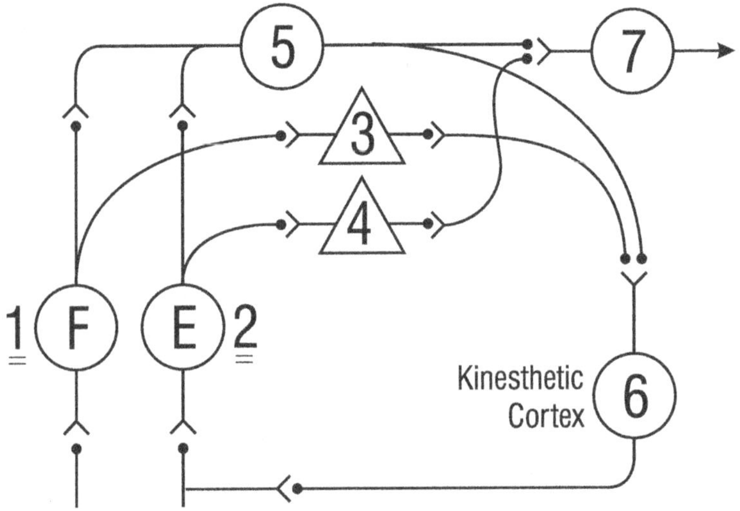

Figure 8: Pulsing Circuit

This circuit has seven neurons. Neurons (3) and (4) are inhibitory, the rest excitatory. The circuit is in the sensorimotor cortex where receptor neurons vary proportionately to varying flexor muscles motor units while receptor extensor muscle antagonist neurons undergo inverse variations. Bioelectric potentials from peripheral muscles are received first by neuron (1) or by neuron (2) but never simultaneously. The axon terminals of neuron (5) – bifurcated from the axonal stem – are the terminals of the circuit. Potentials are routed either through the superior axon collateral of (5) in which case there is activation of neuron (7) – the first neuron of a downstream circuit —; or, through the inferior axon collateral of (5) activating interneuron (6) which, in turn, activates receptor neuron (2). This closes the circuit. Note that neuron (5) activates either (7) thereby activating downstream circuits, or it activates (6) thereby closing the circuit, but never both simultaneously.

Neuron (1) – ("F") – receives potentials from a varying flexor muscle. Neuron (2) – ("E") – receives potentials from the varying extensor antagonist, but fractions of a second after "F." "E" has *two* dendrites, one linked with the (subcortical) extensor muscle, the other receiving potentials of intracortical origin – from interneuron (6) when (6) is activated.

The axons of "F" and "E" are bifurcated. The superior collaterals, longer than the inferior collaterals, each synapse with a dendrite of (5). The inferior (and shorter) axon collaterals of (1) and (2) synapse respectively with inhibitory neurons (3) and (4). The distances between (3), (4) and (5) are less than those between (1), (2) and (5). Therefore if conduction velocities are equal in all parts of the circuit and if activation times of (3) and (4) are negligible, the circuit functions as follows:

Potentials from flexor muscles varying before their extensor antagonists are received by the dendrites of (1), causing it to vary and thus propagate potentials both to (3) which is inhibitory, and to one of the bifurcated dendrites of (5). (5's) axon is also bifurcated, the superior axon terminal synapsing with (7), the inferior with (6). Since the (1)-(3)-(6) distance is shorter than that of (1)-(5), the inhibitory potential from (3) arrives at its synapse with (6) fractionally before the potential from (5) traveling in (5's) inferior axon terminal. Neuron (6) will have been rendered refractory (be inhibited) to excitation by (5). Only (7) – a neuron of a downstream circuit – will be caused to vary by (5) and activation of (1) *always and only* activates (7). Thus, *so long as (1) varies before (2)*, the (5) – (7) synapse (*or relay*) is open, corresponding to a binary 0 – and current potentials) cannot flow from (5) to (6).

When, at the body surface, it is the extensor muscle that varies before its flexor antagonist, the cortical kinesthetic sequence is totally different. (2's) longitudinal dendritic terminal receives potentials from varying extensor muscle motor units. (2) varies, sending potentials in the long dendrite of (5) as well as to inhibitory interneuron (4). (4) is activated, propagating a potential to (7). Since the (2)-(4)-(7) distance is shorter than (2)-(5)-(6), (7) is inhibited and cannot be activated by (5's) superior axon terminal. (5's) inferior axon terminal, however, activates (6) which in turn activates (2) *thus closing the circuit (which pulsates so long as (2) varies before [1])*. Current remains in the circuit, the (5)-(7) relay is closed and this constitutes binary 1. In summary: the (5)-(7) relay is always either open or closed. The functional result is a pulsing circuit, where the open (flexor) state corresponds to binary 0, and the closed (extensor) state to binary 1. Because flexor/extensor muscle couples vary inversely, whenever the (5)-(7) relay is open we have flexion while whenever it is closed we have extension (i.e. binary 1). Finally, relays such as (5)-(7) constitute neuronal switches which are either open or closed and diagrammed previously.

The Half-Adder

If David C Noelle's figure of "about" a thousand synapses per neuron is correct, then switches or relays similar to the 5 – 7 relay described above may be *inputs* to the basic calculation and/or logic circuit of the neuronal computer analogous to manufactured half-adders. A 5 – 7 type relay from an IS-WAS or discriminator circuit is either open (binary 0) or closed (binary 1). But the input of a neuronal half-adder would have to be *two* 5 – 7 type relays, each symbolizing in binary the equivalent of flexor contraction and extensor relaxation (switch open = 0) or the reverse (switch closed = 1). The half-adder totals the fed-in 1's and the 0's by means of AND, OR and NOT gates. Given two 5 – 7 inputs from the kinesthetic cortex, there are four input possibilities:

1. 0+0: both circuits symbolize flexion
2. 1+0: there is extension in the first, flexion in the second
3. 0+1: there is flexion in the first, extension in the second
4. 1+1: both symbolize extension

The hypothetical structuring of neuronal logic gates serving to calculate, reason or both is predicated on the previously described, verified phenomena of neuronal spatial and temporal summation of received potentials. Neurons, it will be recalled, have an excitation threshold. This means that generating potentials of their own requires stimuli (received potentials) of sufficient intensity. In some cases a single received potential might suffice. But when the threshold is high, sufficient stimulation requires one of two excitatory devices, or a combination of both. In spatial summation sufficient stimulation is a product of individual, simultaneous stimuli received in several dendrites of the cell to be activated. Although one or a few simultaneous stimuli are insufficient to trigger a potential, some critical, greater number will do so. In temporal summation, simultaneous stimuli will not trigger activation. Instead, *sequential* stimuli precisely spaced in time are needed. The first stimulus "primes" the neuron. The following stimulus either activates it or primes it further until some succeeding potential produces activation. If the "priming" stimulus or stimuli are not followed by the triggering stimulus within the required time, there will be no activation. These are the proven mechanisms whereby neurons activate each other.

For illustration, I shall describe a neuronal half-adder when the circuit adds 1+1 (possibility number [4] in the previous text). In other words, the two 5 – 7 type relays are both closed signifying binary 1+1 (in the case of kinesthesia, contraction of two motor units of a flexor muscle and relaxation of two motor units of the extensor antagonist): Figure 8.

Now, in binary, the number 2 is symbolized by: 10. Therefore the electric pulse state at the output neurons of the half-adder must "read" 0 for cell #11 and 1 for #15 when the input neurons (#7 relay types) simultaneously symbolize 1 (i.e., 1+1).

Let us postulate an "OR" neuron to have a low stimulation threshold so that activation requires stimulation of just one of many dendrites.

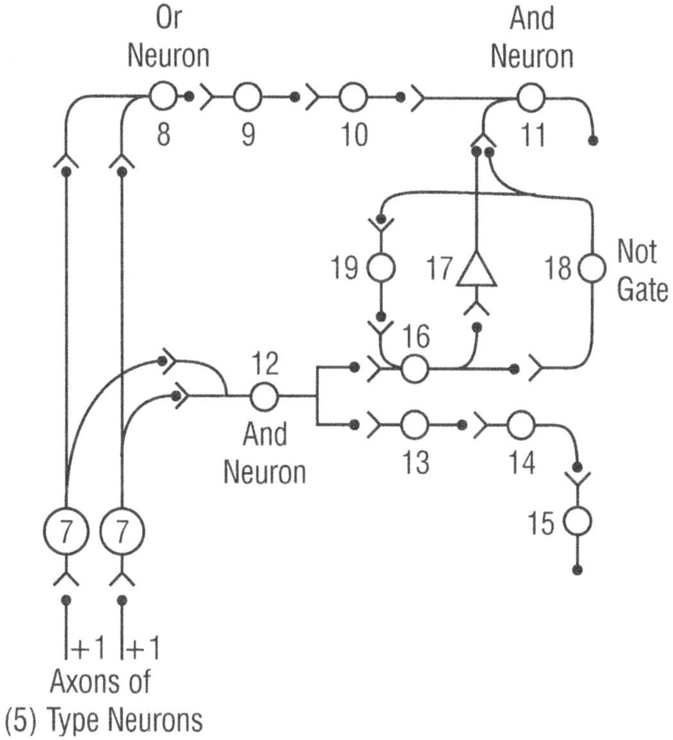

Figure 9: Neuronal Half-Adder

Let us postulate that an AND neuron has a *high* excitation threshold. It is activated *only* when there is temporal summation of stimuli at one or several dendrites, spatial summation by simultaneous stimuli at multiple dendrites or a combination of the two.

And a not *gate* (not neuron!) is an inverter. When its input is 1, its output is 0, and vice-versa. This is realized by the combination of neurons 16, 17, 18 and 19.

Here, then, is how our neuronal half-adder adds an input of two binary 1's furnishing the answer 2 (10 in binary).

The pulsing circuits upstream of both #7-type neurons have opened (signifying binary 1+1 to the half-adders). The axon of each "7" neuron is bifurcated. One axon terminal synapses with one of the two dendrites of the AND neuron (#12), the other axon terminal synapsing with one of the two dendrites of the OR neuron (#8). In reality, if it is true that neurons may synapse with one thousand other neurons, then a realistic diagram would show neurons with considerably more than two dendrites or axons, or axonal and dendritic ramifications into multiple – not merely two – terminals. Axons merely bifurcating and a mere two dendrites per cell are diagrammed for the sake of clarity and simplicity in following the text.

The opening of the two 5 – 7 relays has activated the two 7-type neurons. Both therefore activate the #12 (AND) neuron, which has a high excitation threshold. It varies *because* both of its dendrites received potentials. This AND neuron has a bifurcated axon, so its potential is relayed along the superior axon terminal to neuron #16, and via the inferior axon terminal to neurons 13, 14 and output neuron #15. All neurons in this chain have low excitatory thresholds so that the fact of stimulation of neurons 13 and 14 suffices to elicit +1 at the axon of #15.

The OR neuron (#8) has a low excitation threshold. It is activated because at least one of its dendrites was stimulated. It releases a potential via neurons 9 and 10 to one of the two dendrites of the second AND neuron (#11). This potential arrives simultaneously with that of the inhibitory neuron, #17, at the inferior dendrite of #11. The inhibitory neuron (#17) is an element of the NOT gate, which inverts 1's to 0's and vice versa. It is activated by neuron #16, which is the entry of the NOT gate. Neuron #16 has two dendrites and a bifurcated axon. Its inferior dendrite was stimulated by the superior axon terminal of neuron #12 simultaneously with stimulation of neuron #13 by the inferior axon terminal of #12.

One of neuron #16's axon terminals stimulates the inhibitory neuron (#17) while the other terminal stimulates excitatory neuron #18. The distance between neuron #17 and the inferior dendrite of AND neuron #11 is less than that between neuron #18 and the same dendrite. Therefore there is release of an inhibitory neurotransmitter by #17 at that synaptic junction fractions of a second before the excitatory neurotransmitter of #18. The synapse is refractory to stimulation and since the AND neuron releases potentials only when *both* of its dendrites are stimulated, it is not activated. Therefore the axon terminal of #11 registers 0 at the same time that the terminal of #15 registers 1. We have 10, which is binary 2.

As for the NOT gate: the axon of neuron #18 is bifurcated. When #18 is activated, the excitatory transmitter released at the terminal synapsing with

And neuron #11 is neutralized by the inhibitory transmitter released at the synapse fractionally before by #17. However, the second axon terminal of the bifurcated #18 axon synapses with neuron #19, activating it. Neuron #19 synapses with the second dendrite of #16, forming a closed circuit. So long as neuron #16 is activated by #12 – which, itself is active *only* when *both* #7's are +1 – this closed – circuit ensures that there be *no* stimulation of #11, because there is inhibition at the synapse with 11's inferior dendrite.

Chapter 5: Epilogue

The original version of this manuscript – albeit considerably longer —was finished in 1978. Had it been accepted for publication, I'd have pursued this line of inquiry. But I am 25 years closer to exitus and there are other questions I want to explore, so the follow-up to the theories in this opus will have to be left to others who are inclined to do so.

Neuronal Switches

A neuronal switch would consist of a circuit where an excitatory neuron has a bifurcated axon. Inhibitory neurons act on one or both axonal terminals constituting either a single or a double switch, as follow (Figure 10).

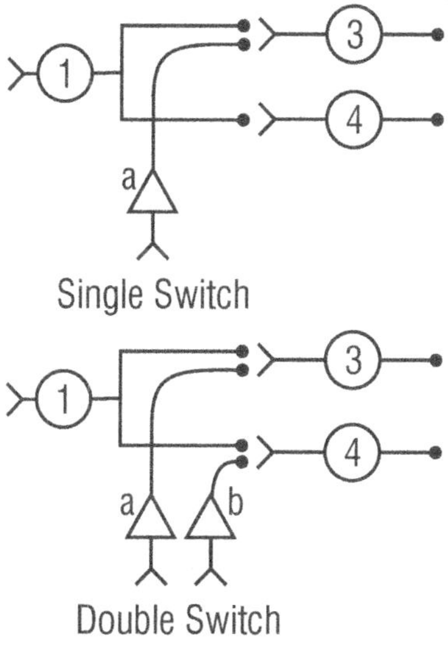

Figure 10: Neuronal Switches

In both switches, neuron (1) is excitatory. The single switch has only one inhibitory neuron, (a), whose single axon synapses with only one of the 1's axon terminals (at the synapse with neuron [3]). Therefore, when (a) is active, conduction to (3) is blocked but not to (4). The double switch has *two* inhibitory neurons. One joins the (1)-(3), and the other the (1)-(4) synapses. When one inhibitory neuron is active, the other is inactive. Therefore, if (a) is active potentials from (1) can activate only (4), and when (b) is active, (1) can activate only (3). Most of the time, the muscles of respiration do their job without conscious effort by the neocortex. The command of respiration is, at these times, autonomic. When we consciously alter our breathing, "I' has become the "pilot." Since "auto" is usually at the control, "auto" is the true pilot and "I" the co-pilot. Or, rather, it is the pilot because in cases of "I"-"auto" contests to control breathing, "auto" always wins – hold your breath the longest you can; if you are not forced to resume breathing before fainting, then you will faint and resume breathing while unconscious. There must, therefore, exist neuronal mechanisms enabling "I" to take control of respiration from "auto," and enabling "auto" to override "I."

The Concept of a Set

"Cantor's definition of a set: A set is the result of collecting together certain well-determined objects of our perception or our thinking into a single whole; these objects are called the elements of the set."

"If an object *a* is an element of a set S, one writes a ∈ S (read 'a belongs to S' or 'S contains a'); one writes a ∉ S if *a* is not an element of S. If S is the set of elements a, b, c, ..., one writes S- {a, b, c...}, for instance, {1, 2,...} is the set of the positive natural numbers. If S contains only one element *a*, then S is called a *singleton*, S – (a)... If S contains two distinct elements a_ and *b*, then S is called an unordered pair, S +-{a, b}."

"A *subset* T of a set is any set whose elements all belong to S; this is denoted by T < S...."

And, "Sets whose elements are themselves sets are called *families* or *systems*..." [9]

"... Much of the work in the sciences relates to data that are functionally related by no known exact formula. In some cases, theoretical considerations dictate the form of the function, in others the data themselves suggest a possible relation; but in many cases there is no hint as to what the relation might be."

"In any event it is desirable to know the form of the exact functional relation, if one exists, or some approximation which will adequately describe the relation for matters of interpolation, extrapolation, etc. The process of finding the equation of a curve which passes through or near the points of a set of paired observations is called *curve fitting*, and the equation of the curve thus fitted is called an *empirical equation*."

"In curve fitting we seek the simplest curve which will reasonably explain the data. We treat four types: *linear*, *parabolic*, *exponential* and *power*."

"The Linear Law. Let the observed data be:

X_1	X_2	X_3	...	X_n
Y_1	Y_2	Y_3	...	Y_n

9. "*The VNR Concise Encyclopedia of Mathematics*," W. Gellert, H. Kustner, M. Hellvic, H. Kastner, Van Nostrand & Reinhold Company, 1977, pp. 320-321

"When plotted on rectangular coordinate paper these points may appear to lie almost on a straight line. A line could be drawn, by sight, that might suffice for rough work, but there are two standard methods for fitting a line to these observations which eliminate the guess work. These are 1. T*he method of averages* and 2. *The method of least.*

1. *The method of Averages.* This process involves dividing the given data into two sets equal or nearly equal in numbers of observations, computing the *average point* for each set, and finding the equation of the line passing through these two average points. If the x's in the first set run from X_1 to X_j the average x for that set is:

$$\frac{X_1 = X_1 + X_2 + \ldots + Xj}{J}$$

The average points are therefore given by (x_1, y_1) and (x_2, y_2) where

$$\frac{X_2 = X_j+1 + X_j+2 + \ldots + X_n}{N\text{-}j}$$

And similarly for the y's." [10]

10. Analytic Geometry, by C.O. Oakley, Barnes & Noble, 1957, p.p. 159-160

Made in the USA
Monee, IL
04 November 2026

67387012R00098